THERAPY AND ETHICS

CURRENT ISSUES IN BEHAVIORAL PSYCHOLOGY

Series Editor

Robert S. Ruskin, Ph.D.

Chairman, Department of Psychology and
Director, Center for Personal Instruction
Georgetown University
Washington, D.C.

Other Books in this Series

The Social Skills Basis of Psychopathology
E. Lakin Phillips, Ph.D.

THERAPY AND ETHICS
The Courtship of Law and Psychology

Norman J. Finkel, Ph.D.
Associate Professor of Psychology
Georgetown University
Washington, D.C.

With an Introduction by
Nicholas N. Kittrie, J.D., LL.M., S.J.D.
Professor of Criminal and Comparative Law
American University Law School
Washington, D.C.

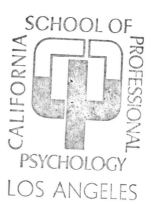

GRUNE & STRATTON
A Subsidiary of Harcourt Brace Jovanovich, Publishers
New York   London   Toronto   Sydney   San Francisco

Grune & Stratton, Inc.
111 Fifth Avenue
New York, New York 10003

Distributed in the United Kingdom by
Academic Press, Inc. (London) Ltd.
24/28 Oval Road, London NW 1

Library of Congress Catalog Number 79-6347
International Standard Book Number 0-8089-1222-4

Printed in the United States of America

To my parents, Max and Dorothy, for compassionately teaching me my first lessons in paternalism, and

To my daughter, Jenny, for imparting bright, new, fresh perspectives on the matter.

I dedicate this book.

Contents

Foreword

Two years ago when I began to think of topics for inclusion in this series, *Current Issues in Behavioral Psychology,* it became apparent that no series of this type would be complete without a thorough exploration of the broad ethical issues facing the behavioral therapist today. Psychology and behavioral science in general have developed techniques for producing change of individual behavior which, if left unchecked, could pose a serious problem to our societal well-being. The therapeutic techniques developed over the past decade are in themselves neither good nor bad and are analogous in a very real sense to another current technology — atomic energy. Therapeutic techniques, as in the case of atomic energy, can be used for obviously unethical or immoral purposes and society, particularly the therapeutic and legal communities, must constantly guard against such excesses in the behavioral domain.

In this book Dr. Finkel has attempted to present the interface between the therapeutic models currently in existence and the legal ramifications of their use. No discussion of therapeutic ethics would be complete without a sound historical perspective, and this also Dr. Finkel admirably supplies. *Therapy and Ethics: The Courtship of Law and Psychology* should prove a useful addition to the libraries of behavioral practitioners and lawyers alike. My personal thanks go to my friend and colleague, Norman Finkel, for writing such a book.

Robert S. Ruskin, Ph.D.

Preface

This work focuses on *therapy* and *ethics*. It starts from the supposition that both must be cultivated for patients and therapists to grow.

The plan is to examine past and current practices in which mental professionals have involved themselves; this covers contractual and involuntary therapy, behavior modification, psychopharmacological treatment, psychosurgery, psychiatric commitment, competency hearings and insanity defenses, predicting dangerousness and mental illness, giving "expert" testimony, and providing institutional treatment. An examination of these topics will lead the reader past the familiar terrain of couches and clients, through cases and courtrooms, to the back wards — and back again. The journey will cross the domains of *psychology, law,* and *ethics.*

Currently, there is much discontent, contention, and paradox in the field of treatment. It is, unfortunately, an all too common sight today for patients to enter the courtroom seeking relief from their healers as well as from their disorders; and therapists, formerly the defenders of mental health, now have to defend themselves and their practices. How is it that our best motivations can spawn the most questionable of practices? And why is it that such formerly lofty words as "paternalism," "benevolence," and "doing good" now have become suspect?

I seek the answers to these questions in our history and in our psychology; I throw in a little mythology as well. The purpose in going back in time to when men of reason first began to "treat" their unreasonable brethren "for their own good" is to explore the psychological roots of helping another. We have not gotten it right yet; the level of criticism and litigation tells us that. Noise signals danger, but may mask answers. I have chosen to penetrate the noise, hoping to find those themes that harmonize our therapy with our ethics. This work quietly makes a few suggestions.

An undertaking like this requires a lot of support. And I have had it. To my colleague and dear friend, Bob Ruskin, who came to me with the idea and faith that I could do it, sincerest thanks. To the publishing team of Grune & Stratton, I am grateful for your patience and support. To my student, Mary Bowman, whose energy, intelligence, and dedication dazzle me, "You're terrific!"

I would like to acknowledge my colleagues at Georgetown who provided guidance through their own writings and timely suggestions: Dan Robinson, Tom Beauchamp, Dan Geller, and Steve Sabat. To friends at the Arlington Day Treatment Center and Mental Health Clinic, who struggle with many of these abstract issues in concrete ways, my thanks for the experiential teachings.

As a psychologist entering a dark legal maze, I needed much navigational aid; my earliest lights were Nicholas Kittrie, Paul Friedman, and Thomas Szasz, whom I thank for their illumination. To Edward Modell and Kenneth Davidson, for keeping me up to date and on my toes, my warmest thanks.

To Claire "fast-fingers" Sabat, for typing and editing, a big hug. And to Georgetown University, for awarding me sabbatical time, a debt of gratitude for the financial and spiritual backing.

Norman J. Finkel, Ph.D.

Introduction

The American people, fervently committed to self-improvement and socioeconomic mobility, have long favored the offerings of popular and applied psychology. How to make friends and influence people, how to reach harmony with one's true self or attain tranquility in the midst of a troubled environment, how to become duly assertive and achieve greater power and success, how to shed offensive character traits and addictions (to substances such as food, alcohol, and tobacco) and acquire more wholesome living habits — these have been and continue to be the dominant concerns of America.

As a consequence, there is probably no other society in which psychological as well as other mental health goals and practitioners play such a prominent role. The fraternity of "treaters" or "therapists" contains scientific experts of various professional stripes, as well as self-proclaimed healers of questionable credentials. Yet despite the tremendous appetite and tolerence displayed by our society towards those who offer their therapeutic wares voluntarily and commercially, there continues a deep and ingrained suspicion of those seeking to impose their healing services upon unwilling clients.

The call for therapeutic services comes from interested individuals as well as from public agencies. A realization of social or psychological inadequacy and desire for self-improvement drives many an individual to seek psychological, psychiatric, or some other form of counseling and curative services. But therapy is often invoked by the police and other governmental organs as a measure of public protection. With regard to both the proven and convicted offender and the mentally abnormal person with a prognosis of potential wrongdoing, the offer of "treatment" or "therapy" seems a most promising antidote. In the traditional arena of criminal justice, rehabilitation has long ago supplanted retribution as a major goal. Psychologists and other mental health practitioners are expected accordingly to furnish the requisite rehabilitative formula. In the related areas of mental illness, juvenile delinquency, drug addition, and alcoholism, the traditional criminal justice formula of conviction and punishment for past conduct has given way to measures borrowed from preventive medicine. Prediction of future danger has been replacing the finding of past criminality, and prevention of future harm is taking the place of punishment. Among those recruited to diagnose the existence and the degree of social and mental deviance and to help determine or predict the potential of future harm, psychologists as well as other behavioral scientists have occupied a prominent place.

For the young mental health practitioner the employment market offers numerous opportunities to serve, not as a private therapist but as the agent of the state. Oftentimes, this practitioner, trained primarily to dispense therapy, is called upon to help decide who is competent to stand trial and who is to be exempted from guilt by reason of insanity. He or she is given charge of the battery of tests to help determine who is mentally ill or mentally retarded, who is an occasional drug abuser and who is an addict, who is a social drinker and who is a chronic alcoholic. The same mental health practitioner, prepared to offer counsel and aid to those seeking it, may become the official gatekeeper for various involuntary confinement and treatment programs. The practitioner prominently aids in deciding who should be confined or treated for society's and his or her own best interests, and who has reached such a state of recovery to justify return to the open community.

As a courtroom witness, as an expert for the state, and as a professional performing administrative functions, the psychologist and his other colleagues in the therapeutic community find themselves possessing important powers of compulsion. How should they exercise these powers? What part should they take in the battle of experts orchestrated by the combatting lawyers? How are they to resolve the conflict between the individual's right to be different versus the state's right to protect and improve itself and its citizens? And equally important: Who is to be viewed as the therapist's client—the patient who may require and sometimes may refuse treatment, or the state that has retained the expert in order to help with the protection of the public interest?

The mental health practitioner's conception of his role is closely interwoven with his own and with the prevailing social and political philosophy. To the adherents of the Hobbesian outlook on the state, the major function of public authority is to prevent men, who differ little from beasts, from harming each other. It is not viewed as the mission of public power to engage in compulsory programs designed to enhance the quality of life. A contrasting perspective is presented by the disciples of John Locke, who urge that society's goal must be the active enhancement of the common good. To the adherents of Locke the unequivocal reply to Cain's rhetorical question is direct: "Yes, Cain, you *are* your brother's keeper!"

By asserting its paternalistic duties and benevolent aims, the modern state has set out to offer not only public welfare to those seeking it, but also to thrust involuntary therapeutic services on unwilling others. At times those subject to state control and sanctions under the claim of *parens patriae* have far exceeded the number of those confined and punished as convicted criminals. Accepting at face value the benevolent assertions of the "therapeutic state," behavioral scientists and other mental health practitioners failed to see their role implications. Responding enthusiastically to the call for public service, the therapists preferred to ignore their own co-option into the system of public controls.

The past two decades have witnessed a growing challenge to the state functioning as therapist. Both legislatures and courts have been called into action. Stringent substantive criteria have been formulated that narrow the categories of those subject to state intervention. New procedural rules have been introduced granting those offered involuntary therapy — juvenile delinquents, drug addicts, alcoholics, and psychopaths — due process safeguards similar to those available to persons charged with crimes. Conditions of confinement and the availability of actual treatment also came under legal scrutiny.

What is unique about Norman Finkel's volume is that it focuses not on the legal, political, or budgetary aspects of the state's venture into therapy. What concerns Finkel most is his role, the role of his discipline, and the role of fellow mental health practitioners in the growing system of public therapy. The volume is well researched and carefully documented. If offers the therapist, of whatever stripe, the opportunity and the tools of professional self-assessment. Norman Finkel is a sensitive practitioner and teacher of psychology. He recognizes the valid criticisms directed towards the functioning of his own and related disciplines. He realizes that legal and other external regulations perform only a limited function, and he seeks to help with the formulation of the therapist's own professional ethics.

Finkel's study is a most timely volume. At present,

"treatment," "therapy," "rehabilitation," and other related public efforts for the improvement of those suffering from vocational, educational, and psychological shortcomings are under great attack. Some critics have proclaimed the total inefficiency of these efforts. Finkel does not accept this nihilistic and unsubstantiated pessimism. He sets out, instead, to bring needed enlightenment to his fellow practitioners and to improve their capacity for service, thereby fostering a system of voluntary services which are not imposed upon but are called for by those in need.

Nicholas N. Kittrie, J.D., LL.M., S.J.D.
American University Law School

THERAPY AND ETHICS

1

The twentieth century mental health professional stands today at
ancient crossroads: his desire to help another individual leads
him to the therapeutic path, yet his "right" to traverse that path
and the "correctness" of that path have been called into question.
Symptomatically, and with increasing frequency, he has been
called into court and called before the court of public opinion, not
so much to defend the defendant, but to defend himself and his
practices. The old adage, "healer heal thyself" is heard again.

So he pauses. And for good reason. The voices calling him
into question come from within the profession as well as from
without and cut across varying ideologies and politics. He is hearing from more than "fringe elements," whose usual utterances
can be taken apart and shrugged off. Now it is eminent spokes-
men in the fields of psychiatry, psychology, law, and ethics, who
are wondering aloud whether the patient needs *protection* from
the healer; and the refrain is getting louder. The therapist is
hearing from another voice too, this one from within: not hallucinations, mind you, but the voice of conscience.

So he pauses to reflect and examine himself and his conduct:
to get himself "straight" before he attempts to straighten another, and to find the "ethical footing" to support his humanitar-
ian desires.

I suggest that if you examine the mental health professional
and his context, if you really pierce the fabric, so to speak, you
will find the mental health professional tied by many threads to
his community, the courts, his profession, his patients, and his
2   beliefs. I am reminded by image of a passage from Freud's *The*

A Tangled Web of
Ethical Threads

Interpretation of Dreams, in which he quotes several lines from Goethe (1967) that translate so:

> . . . a thousand threads one treadle throws,
> where fly the shuttles hither and thither,
> Unseen the threads are knit together,
> And an infinite combination grows.

Goethe, *Faust,* Part I (Scene 4)
(translation by Bayard Taylor)
(p. 317)

Freud found it an appropriate image for dreams, and I for the waking reality of the mental health professional. More and more the "community of reasonable men seek the professional out as emissary to their "unreasonable brethren." As Michel Foucault (1973) has written in a powerful work, *Madness and Civilization: A History of Insanity in the Age of Reason,* "In the serene world of mental illness, modern man no longer communicates with the madman: on one hand, the man of reason delegates the physician to madness, thereby authorizing a relation only through the abstract universality of disease . . ." (p. x).

"The abstract universality of disease," however, is affecting communities in very *concrete* ways: there is the visible and saddening waste of human potential; there are anxiety, depression, and problems of alcohol and addiction that leave scars on arms, families, and communities; there is the economic waste of people too troubled to work, and the economic burden of those who have to support them; and there is the fear of this "other," this   3 "strange" stranger in our midst, our "kin but not our kind," who spurs the community of reasonable men to action. The community of reasonable men, seeking answers and safety, pulls the thread that ties them to the mental health professional and, through him, seeks to affect their unreasonable brethren. If only Cain and Abel had a therapist.

Another thread knits families to the mental health professional. Families, functioning families, are cornerstones of psychological health. Professionals are already quite familiar with the staggering amount of correlational evidence linking broken and troubled families to psychological disturbances in its members. Almost every disorder in any abnormal psychology text or in any Diagnostic and Statistical Manual (DSM-I, II, or III) finds a corresponding theory and correlative facts that joint to family etiology. When a family in crisis calls a mental health professional, they usually find a receptive ear. "Our son is sick." "Our daughter needs therapy." "Our father is drunk again, and dangerous." "Our mother is depressed, and speaks of ending it." The professional listens. Often, however, he is asked to act. "Treat her." "Hospitalize him." "Give her shock therapy, or something." "Make him take his medication." If he takes action on behalf of the troubled family, he may put himself in opposition with the family's "troubled" member; a likely consequence of this is that the "therapeutic" relationship with the "troubled" member becomes an *adversary* relationship rather than an *alliance*. A likely consequence of that is reduced effectiveness. Although jeopardizing the therapeutic relationship and defeating its effectiveness are surely technical issues of concern, what can we say regarding the professional's conduct—his ethics? Should he get involved? And if so, to what extent? Are the family threads about to tie him into knots?

Another thread links marriage to the mental health professional. One volume of the Joint Commission Report on Mental Illness and Health surveyed Americans regarding their health, happiness, and professional contact (Gurin, Veroff, & Feld, 1960); when they surveyed those who had gone for help, the problem area most frequently cited was, "Spouse; marriage." So when husbands and wives call the mental health professional regarding trouble with their marriage, and the evidence indicates that they do call, the professional listens. But should he act, and if so, how? What if he is asked to aid in the involuntary commitment of one party? What if he is asked to give testimony as to the *mental competency* or *potential dangerousness* of a spouse? Threads that can ally him to one member are often the very same threads that alienate him from the other.

As psychiatry and psychology have grown, so has the respect afforded them. As Perry London (1964) writes in *The Modes and Morals of Psychotherapy,* "Its professors and practitioners, once contemptuously regarded as eccentrics mumbling arcane obscenities at the fringe of medicine, have advanced from relative obscurity to chairs of eminence and couches of opulence in the finest universities and neighborhoods in the Western World" (p. v).

Contrary opinions also exist. Some see psychiatry (a) on the decline, (b) as despotism in the name of health, (c) in depression and on the couch, (d) dying, and (e) already dead. Thomas Szasz (1963), in *Law, Liberty, and Psychiatry,* sounded some of the earliest warning signals that the discipline of psychiatry was in trouble: "in trouble" precisely because it was advancing unthinkingly, in part, and in part because it was advancing under the banner of certain mental health euphemisms that masked a type of despotism and a "tyranny of therapy." By offering safety, security, and the mirage of mental health while practicing social engineering, Szasz saw psychiatry running risks of infringing on liberty.

Another view of psychiatry was featured on the cover of *Time* magazine (April 2, 1979), under the banner "Psychiatry's Depression." The article was entitled "Psychiatry on the Couch," and it portrayed psychiatry in its middle years, in acute depression, in crisis over its own identity, and struggling with its delusions of grandeur and declining abilities to cope.

E. Fuller Torrey (1974) announced that psychiatry was dying in *The Death of Psychiatry;* whether or not "reports of the death" or the book's title were, or are, premature, Torrey's first recommendation was to hold an Irish wake for psychiatry.

Whether psychiatry is a super nova or a white dwarf, advancing or declining, in good health or ill, is under debate today. The recent Report to the President in *The President's Commission on Mental Health* (1978) can be viewed not only as a survey of mental health in America, but as an examination of the health of the mental health professions. The time for temperature taking is at hand.

One area that has heated up and grown over the years is the interface of law and psychology. The court's reliance on the mental health professional has increased. As Robinson (1973) writes, "There is a conspiracy of success: . . . that form of humanistic thought that weds the courts to the treatment centers is in the ascendant . . ." (p. 129). Where past punishments have failed to control crime and change the criminal and where punishment seems to be an "inappropriate" response (i.e., punishing someone who is sick), the courts have turned increasingly from punishment to "treatment." As one illustration out of many of this view, I cite the words of Justice Stewart, speaking for the Court in *Robinson* v. *California*:[1]

> But, in the light of contemporary human knowledge a law which made a criminal offense of such a disease (mental illness) would doubtless be universally thought to be an infliction of cruel and unusual punishment in violation of the Eighth and Fourteenth Amendments. . . . Even one day in prison would be a cruel and unusual punishment for the "crime" of having a common cold. (p. 763)

The threads wedding the courts to the mental health professional increase and grow tighter. One example of this is in the area of crime.

Crime statistics are rising according to yearly police and FBI accounts. Maybe more importantly, however, crime "seems" to be inexorably rising, heightening fears in an already alarmed citizenry. Perhaps the *psychological* reality is far more important than the *factual* reality, with *perceptions* closer to the "heart and soul" of the matter than objective rates of rising crime. We *may* have a real and growing problem with crime; what is far more *certain* is that we have a *psychological* problem with crime. Our fears provide us with visceral documentation.

Our fears, however, are not uniform across criminal offenses. Some acts seem so offensive, so "out of the ordinary" and disturbing, that many laymen, media editorialists, judicial authorities, legislators, and mental health professionals suggest that they must be the product of a "disturbed" mind. These "offensive" offenses are not necessarily the most brutal, nor the crimes usually punished by the harshest sentences: premeditated murder, for example, in the case of someone murdering another to obtain financial gain, although not condoned, can, at least, be well *understood*. In short, we understand the *motivation*. Thus, although the act of premeditated murder does not engender our sympathy, the "greed" motivating the murder in the above example does find its likeness (and perhaps sympathy) in our own, "all too human" side; but "offensive" offenses are another matter. When we first hear of crimes such as mass murder, "random" and "unpremeditated" murders (and here I think of Jules Fieffer's chilling, black-comedy, *Little Murders*), molestations of small children, rape, incest, and homosexual assault, these acts leave an incredulous look on our faces that *understanding* is often una-

---

[1] *Robinson* v. *California* 370 U. S. 660.

ble to erase. Enmity, not sympathy, is likely to be the aroused sentiment.

A case in point, quoted from Nicholas Kittrie's (1971) *The Right to Be Different,* is the following:

> In 1957 two young boys were sexually assaulted and killed in a park south of Boston, Massachusetts. The person charged with the crime had only months before been released from prison after serving a sentence for another sexual offense. The Massachusetts Legislature immediately reacted by enacting a Sexually Dangerous Law which is still in effect. Under this statute, persons convicted of sexual offenses may be committed for indeterminate treatment, from one day to life, to a "hospital," in lieu of a criminal proceeding and incarceration. (p. 176)

We now treat this crime and criminal differently from other crimes and criminals. Indeed, we "treat" rather than punish, sending them off to "hospitals" rather than prisons.

Why this discrimination in law? When Justice is supposedly "blind," how is it she can "see" differences? What reasons, with what ethical underpinnings, support Justice's "sight" — and "our conduct" — conduct that undercuts the *equal protection* safeguards of the constitution? These, and other questions, will be pursued in full later in the text. For now, let me draw the health professional deeper into this story, at least to anticipate, if not deepen, the ethical dilemmas that lie ahead.

Returning to the Massachusetts legislature and the passage of the Sexually Dangerous Law, we know that their constituency was alarmed. Legislators, wishing to assuage the fear and ensure their future, were predisposed to act; yet testimony and evidence were needed to support the different treatment of "these" offenders. Are "they" different from "us"? It is here that the mental health professional is likely to enter this drama, invited to provide *expert* answers, while not slipping on any ethical issues — a neat trick. Later, when the law is in place and operational, he may be called into court, as an expert witness, to give testimony as to the "saneness" of a defendant to stand trial, or if that defendant does stand trial, to give testimony as to the "sanity" of the act and the actor. Ascending still further along the road that leads from courts to treatment centers, the professional may be asked to cure his "committed charge" — to walk a therapeutic tightrope on an ethical leg. The question here is one of balance.

The mental health professional stands within the context of his own discipline, a discipline that has grown in size, prestige, and impact, but which now groans from past and current strains.

Looking backward, the discipline's history is checkered with questionable practices. Historical brutalities have been recorded (Deutsch, 1949; Foucault, 1973) on paper and in our conscience. Our past omissions and failings no doubt have an effect on present practices, perhaps like the collective unconscious affecting conscious actions, in a *compensatory* way. Thus we seek to atone and make restitution: we seek to produce a healthy society. In this light (but not solely in this light) the "community mental health" and "community psychology" movements provide interesting current examples (Cowen, 1973; Hobbs, 1964) of closer and deeper professional involvement in community life.

The new community psychologist is asked to be an active participant in the problems of society (Rappaport, 1977), rather than maintaining the passive–receptive stance of an age just passing. He is asked to be a "social change agent," a "mental health quarterback," a "social engineer," a "participant–conceptualizer," and a "political activist" (Bennett, Anderson, Cooper, Hassol, Klein, & Rosenblum, 1966; Cowen, 1967). As the professional attempts to intervene earlier in problems rather than belatedly, as he attempts to *detect* disorders at their earliest stages and *prevent* them from worsening, or prevent them from occurring at all, he runs grave ethical risks of doing too much, and of intruding too far on rights that are properly left to the individual. It seems fortunate that these value-laden issues are receiving greater attention (Rappaport, 1977); they are only mentioned here as one more sticky thread that can ensnare the helper in an ethical web.

Standing, sitting, or lying before the "troubled" mental health professional is a "troubled" individual, or an individual who "troubles" significant others (e.g., family, schools, courts, police). What do we call him? How do we *see* him? Is he our brother, or the "other"? "Conflicted," "sick," "a client," "patient," or "child"? Which is he? In this case the words matter; for what we call him tells us something about how we *see* him. Our words come to mirror our own *perceptions,* and the helper's perceptions of the helpee tie him to certain actions and options. If you *see* the person as responsible for his own actions, different consequences follow than if you do not. If you *see* the chronological adult as a "psychological child" rather than as an adult, other consequences follow. What you can do, or may wish to do for another, is balanced by what we ought to do, or are allowed to do. Yet the balance point slides, as the history of "therapeutic incursions" reveal (Foucault, 1973). In our contemporary time a therapeutic attitude has replaced earlier epochs of cruelty and neglect (Kittrie, 1971; Szasz, 1970). In our own enlightenment we seek to assist and improve the lot of psychologically troubled individuals; yet this often gets us into more trouble. Our incursions, now being beneficent rather than malevolent, only cloud and complicate this delicate balancing of rights. It is easy to reject malevolent interventions; but when the helper "only wishes to help," protestations are more difficult to formulate and resistances are less effective.

It is to these "difficult to formulate" issues, that this book is chiefly addressed. Thus, when speaking about therapist–patient interactions, I will be confining myself, in the main, to interactions motivated by the *best* intentions of the therapist. This is not, in any way, a denial of historical or current misuses and abuses of therapy, nor is it a denial that malevolent, incompetent, neglectful, or uncaring therapists exist. Rather, it is just that in balancing, on the one hand, society's right to protect itself and improve itself against the individual's right to be different and to be left alone, the most interesting and difficult choices seem to arise when both parties believe in the wisdom of their respective positions, and their ethical underpinnings.

This "threadbare" tale and metaphor would be incomplete without mentioning our "heart strings." The good therapists, to whom this work is pointed, bring to their work and their clients a certain *heart-felt* attitude that threads through their being. Call it "altruism," "humanitarianism," "a caring," or "a desire to help another," we all have it in varying doses or we would not be in the business. It may be, if you believe certain process and outcome studies of the effectiveness of psychotherapy (Urban & Ford, 1971), that this very attitude is the essential active ingredient in our helping. In short, therapy may work, when it works, because of this helping attitude. Yet this very same attitude may be the source of therapy's failure. I am reminded of the comments of Freud and Menninger, two eminent analysts, regarding the therapist's sympathy, caring, and giving. Freud, in his 1912 paper, "Recommendations for Physicians on the Psychoanalytic Method of Treatment" (1924) urged that the therapist put "aside all his own feelings, including that of human sympathy" (p. 329), in performing his therapeutic function; and Menninger (1958), in his *Theory of Psychoanalytic Technique,* tells us not to rush to *give* our patients interpretations—that sometimes we must give by *not* giving.

This lesson was brought home in the following, personal anecdote. When my daughter was four years old, she openly expressed the desire to ride a two wheeler. This touched my memories of when my father taught me to ride a bike. I had been waiting for this time. I had had many anticipatory fantasies of this special joy of fatherhood – teaching your kid how to ride a bicycle. I had even thought of specific techniques – clear improvements on my father's teaching – that I wanted to try out. I could help her with her fear of falling, support her courage, and so on. These were *my desires* to help. Imagine my feelings when she called me outside the house to show me "something": she had been secretly practicing on a neighbor's two wheeler for the past four days, and when I came outside, she rode by, beaming.

As for me, there was confusion. I was happy for her and *her* accomplishment, but sad that I did not get to help in the process. My best paternalistic desires were unfulfilled. Yet her independence, initiative, persistence, and *self*-direction were my deepest hopes for her – the "end point" of my paternalism, so to speak. She had just beaten me to it, finding her own help rather than mine. And that is the moral of many a therapeutic story: sometimes the therapist's heart strings must be broken and put aside if the client is to take responsibility and grow.

The web of threads has now been spun. Like a spider trying to read his "signal thread," the one that discriminates signal from noise, we will search for those clear ethical signals and precepts to guide our conduct and secure our footing. First, however, some more noise.

THE TECHNIQUES OF THERAPY

Psychotherapy's "roots" are steeped in history and lodged within the archetypal patterns of our collective unconscious (Finkel, 1976); temporally speaking, twentieth century psychotherapy's more immediate predecessor could be seen in the late eighteenth century practice of "mesmerism"; spatially speaking, or at least from the view of the psychoanalytic couch, the unseen face of Anton Mesmer could be "seen" behind the unseen face of Sigmund Freud. As history records, Mesmer and mesmerism drew mixed revues: "bravos" from the Paris court and the ladies with "Maladie d'amour or melancholie erotique,"[2] but "boos" and skepticism from the Académie des Sciences (Zilboorg & Henry, 1941). This roughly paralleled the reception of Freud and Freudianism, when his person and views hit the American shore: "kudos" from sprouting Psychoanalytic Institutes and Park Avenue patients, but "knowing snickers" and skepticism from budding Behavior-

---

[2] The title of a Jacques Ferrand book, cited by Foucault, 1973.

ists and flowering "Functionalists." For on this side of the Atlantic, the Behaviorists were cultivating in rich soil, and at their hands there flourished more certain, and more powerful, techniques. Although mesmerism and psychotherapy offered insights and glimpses into "the unconscious," they nevertheless had difficulty producing cures—at least at the level that could be consumed by the impatient masses.

Mesmerism died, but hypnosis lived; it spread from Mesmer in Paris to Braid in Manchester, Esdaile in India (by way of London), Grimes in New England, and the Marquis of Puysegur in France (Bernheim, 1947; Erickson, Hershman, & Secter, 1961). In its spread, hypnosis caught the imagination of many, and even "threatened," for a trancelike moment, to deliver the alchemist's and philosopher's Rosetta stone. More often, however, what it did deliver were "gems," which, upon assay, were more apt to be pyrite—"fools gold." Behaviorism minded a surer commodity. Novelists, futurists, science-fiction writers, screenplay writers, and made for TV movie creators, all who speculate in the commodities market, were inventing and reaping more from *behaviorism* too.

In 1931 Aldous Huxley wrote *Brave New World* (1932) and in 1948 George Orwell projected *1984* (1949). In 1958 Aldous Huxley came back for a second look (*Brave New World Revisited,* 1965), and he saw measures of *control* growing in both efficiency and employment, such that "freedom" seemed perched, ever more precariously, on the brink. From the dogs of Pavlov, the white rabbits of Albert, and the rats and pigeons of Skinner came news of more powerful conditioning procedures. Behaviors could be "shaped up" with undergraduate ease; schedules of reinforcement gave predictable responding, at rates the predictor desired; and long chains of responses could be linked together for both comical and serious ends. The "luckless" contender to all this seemed to be "autonomous man."[3]

For all these many years, the only real contender has been *autonomous man* whose demise is at once the necessary and the sufficient condition for the success of behaviorism and its signal patron.

The metaphor of the contest may be too courtly for modern taste but it is hardly reckless. It is ably defended by Skinner, himself, who has assessed the cost of adopting his perspective:

Is man then "abolished"? Certainly not as a species or as an individual achiever. It is the autonomous inner

---

[3] See Robinson, D.N. "Autonomous Man: Are Reports of His Death Exaggerated?"

man who is abolished, and that is a step forward. (Skinner, 1971 p. 205)

This is spirited talk; some might even call it bold. It is not, however, new talk for, as early as page 3 of his *Behavior of Organisms* (1938), actually the first page of the text, he had sounded the same trumpet:

> In more advanced systems of behavior, the ultimate direction and control have been assigned to entities placed within the organism and called psychic or mental. Nothing is gained by this stratagem because most, if not all, of the determinative properties of the original behavior must be assigned to the inner entity, which becomes, as it were, an organism in its own right.

These two quotations are taken from works separated by 33 years, a display of consistency almost without precedent in a world judged to be so fast-changing.

The pace is fast changing: from the 1938 to the 1971 quote, Skinnerian principles and practices have moved from university laboratories to prisons, back wards, and classrooms: children and adults have superseded the rat and pigeon, while token economies, controlled environments, and contingency management have replaced antedated and uncertain measures of control. Techniques of behavior control have grown out of its infancy and into an applied stage, but I maintain that age of enlightenment is not yet at hand.

In 1958, Huxley wrote that "Orpheus has entered into an alliance with Pavlov—the power of sound with the conditioned reflex" (Huxley, 1965 p. 54). In 1973 Robinson cautions us regarding an alliance "of sorts" between neobehaviorism and physiological psychology:

> Two fields that, for so long, coexisted in a most unsteady peace. For decades, the former conducted its affairs with a mythical "empty organism, confident that a natural science of psychology could blossom without the nurturing and protective influences of biology. Concurrently, physiological psychology continued to multiply its reflex units, satisfied that, with enough electrode placements and the right parameters of stimulation, goal-oriented chains of behavior would appear. The undeniable successes of the behavioristic perspective led to the seemingly axiomatic conclusion that psychol-

ogical man is nothing but behavior, while data drawn from "neuropsychology" rendered psychological man nothing but a neural outcome.

Predictably, the two schools met in the limbic system. (p. 130)

They also met in prisons and hospitals, in search of the limbic system of a prisoner or patient that needed "fine tuning": if you were the "searcher," it was called "psychosurgery." According to a U. S. Department of Health, Education and Welfare release, "Psychosurgery: Perspective on a Current Issue" (Brown, Wienckowski, & Bivens, 1973), "Psychosurgery can be defined as surgical removal or destruction of brain tissue or the cutting of brain tissue to disconnect one part of the brain from another with the *intent of altering behavior.* Usually it is performed in the absence of direct evidence of existing structural disease or damage in the brain" (p. 1). The technique is used to control a "variety of emotional and aggressive behaviors"; where, then, would you find a better place than mental hospitals and prisons to test this "current" idea and technique?

Can the patient decline such an offer of "help"? This question and a host of ethical issues were raised in *Kaimowitz and John Doe* v. *Department of Mental Health for the State of Michigan* (Civil Action No. 73-19434-AW, in the Circuit Court for Wayne County. Of note now is the growth of the technique, its potency, and its refinements. Psychosurgery grew out of the lobotomy, which, in turn, grew out of trephining (Finkel, 1976), which is discussed in the following passage:

Newer expulsive techniques were needed. Trephining provided one answer. For some reason, the normal apertures appeared insufficient or inadequate for the demon to escape through, so a new hole was created — usually in the top of the head. This barbaric insult, made by an early "neurosurgeon," was accomplished with a Stone Age tool — the pointed rock — as well as a few able bodies to hold the victim down securely. (The Smithsonian Institution houses both tools and the skulls that have survived from primitive skull surgery.)

Curiously, the treatment survived perhaps because the patient did, too, often enough. (p. 13)

The technique not only survived, it improved. "The pointed rock gave way to the trephining knife — the Peruvian *tumi,* a bronze scalpel which allowed the Incan skull surgeon to make far more elegant and varied cuts. Crosshatching replaced smashing as the mode of entry. The handles of the *tumi* often featured an *intaglio* which showed the procedure in action. The patient, the attendant holding the patient, and the surgeon holding the knife were illustrated on the handle" (Finkel, 1976, p. 14) — a clear case of technical and aesthetic advancement.

The lobotomy offered newer breakthroughs. When the Portuguese neurologist and neurosurgeon, Moniz, received the Nobel Prize in physiology and medicine in 1949, it was for introducing the prefrontal lobotomy into psychiatry in 1935 (Szasz, 1973). Moniz's thinking was to knock out "a small *circle of ideas* which overrule all others and keep recurring in their diseased brain."[4] Moniz did not intrude into brain and person lightly, or whimsically, but after "more than two years of meditation": "My purpose being to annihilate a great number of associations, I preferred to attack (en masse) the cell-connecting fibres of the anterior portion of both frontal lobes aiming at positive results. The method of destruction employed at first was alcohol injections followed by incisions with the leucotome, a small apparatus designed by us for this purpose" (p. 159). This leucotome, or knife, was inserted, through small round holes cut in the skull near the temple, into the white matter of the brain, and then twisted to sever the many connections (Kittrie, 1971, p. 305–306). Techniques improved: the transorbital lobotomy "in which an ice-picklike instrument inserted into the brain through the eye socket is used to cut the frontal lobes," improved the aesthetics, lowered the fatality rate, and reduced undesirable side effects like partial paralysis, loss of bladder control, and convulsions" to more "acceptable," though not perfect, levels. Brown et al. (1973) sum up the development:

> Ever since the first "radical" lobotomies were performed . . . in which virtually all of the subcortical connections of the frontal lobe were severed, surgeons have attempted to refine the techniques to limit the brain destruction in the hope of reducing adverse side effects. . . .
>
> This search for limitation of destruction of brain tissue (and presumably of adverse side effects) culminated in stereotaxic techniques in which a small electrode is positioned in the brain. Geometric coordinates and x-ray inspection are used to place the electrode in a precise location and then the tissue is destroyed at the electrode tip by passing a current through the electrode. With the development of stereotaxic techniques, structures deep within the brain became accessible for destruction, and amygdalotomy, thalamotomy, and hypothalamotomy began to replace lobotomy as psychosurgical procedures. (p. 1)

---

[4] Szasz, 1973, quoting from Egas Moniz, *How I Came to Perform Prefrontal Leucotomy*, Congress of Psychosurgery (Lisboa: Edicoes Atica, 1948) pp. 7–18.

The techniques work "better and better." It is precisely because they work so well that the ethical issues become more acute. The words of Robinson (1973) are instructive:

Psychosurgery is performed in the absence of any collection of ideas warranting the name *theory,* and the methods of behavior modification are applied with increasing vigor and freedom despite their origins in a body of knowledge that has been guided by a self-consciously atheoretical perspective for 40 years. In other words, these therapeutic regimens are adopted not because they spring from theoretically rich, rational, and unsuccessfully challenged expositions, but because *they work.* And, if the relevant literature is to be believed, they work very, very well. Where the hopeful patient once entered (voluntarily) the ambiance of orthodox Freudian treatment with little a priori reason to anticipate a "cure," the modern patient is sent to a far more certain fate. At this point, we are forced to confront an overwhelming ethical issue. While the respective bodies of knowledge do not rest on a theoretical substructure, their implicit hypothesis is that psychological man is *only* behavior or a neural outcome. If we accept this assertion, then the correlated therapies constitute a veritable execution of the person being replaced. This is, of course, too strong — although consistent with the rhetoric — but it does point to the issue. *If we now have therapeutic methods for imposing transformations on psychological man, then our right to apply these methods is bounded.* It is bounded on one side by the legal force of those guarantees against cruel and *unusual* punishment and on the other side by the moral force entailed in respect for the right to be different. (p. 131)

Psychopharmacology, that discipline that studies "the utilization of drugs in restoring or maintaining mental health and for exploring the mind" (Caldwell, 1970, p. 3), has grown enormously in power, influence, and dollars. The tranquilizer, introduced in a major way in the 1950s, is credited with producing a revolution in mental hospital discharges. In 1967, tranquilizers sold at a rate of 95 billion pills per year (Kittrie, 1971). The age of "chemical persuasion," an age that Huxley (1965) fantasized about, is here.

In the Brave New World of my fable there was no whiskey, no tobacco, no illicit heroin, no bootlegged cocaine. People neither smoked, nor drank, nor sniffed, nor gave themselves injections. Whenever anyone felt depressed or below par, he would swallow a tablet or two of a chemical compound called soma. The original soma, from which I took the name of this hypothetical drug, was an unknown plant (possibly *Asclepias acida*) used by the ancient Aryan invaders of India in one of the most solemn of their religious rites. The intoxicating juice expressed from the stems of this plant was drunk by the priests and nobles in the course of an elaborate ceremony. In the Vedic hymns we are told that the drinkers of soma were blessed in many ways. Their bodies were strengthened, their minds were enlightened and in an immediate experience of eternal life they received the assurance of their immortality. But the sacred juice had its drawbacks. Soma was a dangerous drug — so dangerous that even the great sky-god, Indra, was sometimes made ill by drinking it. Ordinary mortals might even die of an overdose. But the experience was so transcendently blissful and enlightening that soma drinking was regarded as a high privilege. For this privilege no price was too great.

The soma of Brave New World had none of the drawbacks of its Indian original. In small doses it brought a sense of bliss, in larger doses it made you see visions and, if you took three tablets, you would sink in a few minutes into refreshing sleep. And all at no physiological or mental cost. The Brave New Worlders could take holidays from their black moods, or from the familiar annoyances of everyday life, without sacrificing their health or permanently reducing their efficiency.

In the Brave New World the soma habit was not a private vice; it was a political institution, it was the very essence of the Life, Liberty and Pursuit of Happiness guaranteed by the Bill of Rights. But this most precious of the subjects' inalienable privileges was at the same time one of the most powerful instruments of rule in the dictator's armory. The systematic drugging of individuals for the benefit of the State (and incidentally, of course, for their own delight) was a main plank in the policy of the World Controllers. The daily soma ration was an insurance against personal maladjustment, social unrest and the spread of subversive ideas. Religion, Karl Marx declared, is the opium of the people. In Brave New World this situation was reversed. Opium, or rather soma, was the people's religion. (pp. 68–69)

The drugs are getting more powerful, even if their action is still "not well understood." In addition to the major and minor tranquilizers, there are mood elevators to stimulate the depressed and antipsychotic agents to reduce delusional thoughts and eliminate hallucinations. Pharmaceutical salesmen, representing a billion-dollar industry, bombard psychiatrists and doctors with ads, sales pitches, free samples, and desk calendars, all in the hope that their brand will be tried. If unpleasant side effects arise, the company is likely to have a second pill, side-effect medication, to offer the physician to offer to his patient.

What if the patient declines to take his medication? What if he says or "acts out" a "no thank you" to this psychopharmacological form of control? Can he be made to take his medicine? As the "controls" get better, as their therapy becomes more potent and visible to courts, doctors, and parents, so do the pressures to use them — even against the objections of the recipient.

Brainwashing, a term made popular following the Korean War, had been used on military prisoners who were subjected to stress techniques aimed at changing their beliefs. This extreme form of coercive persuasion, although not uniformly effective, nonetheless had an impact on a small few. The war ended, but not the controversy about brainwashing. In more recent years, the possibility of brainwashing has been raised in several interesting and diverse cases: It was raised by the defense in the Patricia Hearst case as a way of accounting for the sudden change in attitude and behavior of an upper class, conservative young lady; it was raised in the murder trial of Ronny Zamora, where "TV Intoxication" — television's violence and repeated doses of violence — was linked "subliminally" to the admitted murder committed by a 15-year-old boy (Washington Post, September 30, 1977, p. A11); and it has been raised by parents to account for the sudden conversion and influence of their offspring by certain religious groups, and used, in turn, by some of these same parents to support their attempts to decondition, deprogram, or brainwash back, their "altered" child.

Conditioning, psychosurgery, psychopharmacology, and persuasion have all grown in efficiency, variety, and danger: history illustrates that plowshares can turn into swords, and tools, even *therapeutic* tools, can become weapons. What makes the danger clear, present, and more troubling is the increase in the "applicability" of these tools to present-day psychological and behavioral problems at a pace that outraces the related, ethical discussion. Robinson (1973) warns that, "The greatest danger is that the public will think we know what we are doing instead of appreciating the experimental nature of our enterprise" (p. 133). He suggests that we may have to "curry a bad press," to increase "skepticism and criticism in our recent benefactors, the media," slow the rush to apply, and increase the dialogue among thoughtful men about their ethics and actions.

The therapeutic tool becomes a special thread that runs through this work: it becomes the tightrope upon which therapists must stand and cross. Providing the balance is *ethics,* the study of the therapist's conduct and crossing. This book is a chronical of conduct and crossings, of falls, leanings, and equilibrium. May it be balanced.

2

A man in his late twenties "hangs out" inside and outside an all-night drugstore. He is disheveled in appearance, wears no socks, and his clothes are dirty. It is rumored that he was, or is, a mental patient.

Oh yes, he glares. Some customers feel that he has a menacing look, while others do not notice, or "pay him no mind."

Sometimes he mumbles. Sometimes, when people pass by or avoid him, he talks to himself or the void around him. Occasionally he utters an obscenity directed to no one in particular, although some who hear it are offended.

When spoken to, he may answer, or then again, he may not. When asked, "Why do you stand there?," he answers, "It's a free country." He points to a tattered copy of the United States Constitution, which he carries in his back pocket, a remnant from a junior high school civics class, but which now doubles for a sun visor or umbrella, depending on climate and season.

18   Although there is good agreement among observers that he is

A Hypothetical Case:
The Individual's Right to
Be Different versus The
State's Right to Protect
and Improve Itself

different, there is less agreement as to whether he is dangerous. Although he stares, glares, and may look menacing, he makes no overt threats. Nevertheless he offends some portion of the community, maybe even a significant portion: in a literal and aesthetic way, our eyes, ears, and nose may be affected; in a moral way, our sense of values may be jostled. Yet he lays no hand on us. The question is, "May we lay hands on him?" He does not prevent people from shopping or walking past him. May we prevent him from occupying his square of sidewalk?

This Dickensian character, out of place and era, stands before us today much as he stood in Dickens' time. In fact, one can almost hear the echoes from that earlier Age of Reason. If we listen to those echoes and return to that time, we would probably discover that our hypothetical character was carted off from his corner and confined in a house of correction or Hôspital Général. This was the dumping place for vagrants, mendicants, prodigal sons and spendthrift fathers, blasphemers, libertines, and the insane (Foucault, 1973). These were the forms of unreason that caused offense, shame, dishonor, and scandal; and confinement was sanctioned as a reasonable means to avoid such scandal. When it came time to balancing the "right of families seeking to escape dishonor" against the individual's "right to be left alone," individual liberty came up short. Foucault writes (1973),

> Confinement hid away unreason, and betrayed the shame it aroused; but it explicitly drew attention to madness, pointed to it. . . . But at the same time it assigned to this same madness a special sign: not that of sickness, but that of glorified scandal. Yet there is nothing in common between this organized exhibition of madness in the eighteenth century and the freedom with which it came to light during the Renaissance. In the Renaissance, madness was present everywhere and mingled with every experience by its images or its dangers. During the classical period, madness was shown, but on the other side of bars; if present, it was at a distance, under the eyes of a reason that no longer felt any relation to it and that would not compromise itself by too close a resemblance. Madness had become a thing to look at: no longer a monster inside oneself, but an animal with strange mechanisms, a bestiality from which man had long since been suppressed. (p. 70)

Jumping back to our present time and place, changes have occurred. Across the Atlantic, in a country that fought for liberty and was founded upon liberty, the guarantees of freedom are stronger, and the safeguards against their abridgement are surer. The modern court is less likely to be persuaded by arguments based on "shame," "dishonor," or "scandal," feeling that the price we pay for our pluralism and freedom includes occasional upsets to our sensibilities, although not to our person.

But what if the argument changes? What if the community, family, storekeeper, or shopper no longer argues that their sensibilities, good name, or honor are being harmed, but that an intervention (e.g., a confinement) may *help* the victim? Regarding our Dickensian character, the argument now shifts to *his* best interests, rather than our own — or so it seems.

The best judge of a person's best interests, of course, is usually the person himself. At least "we" would claim that in our own case. Yet there are mitigating circumstances in which this assumption has been challenged successfully. As an example, in our hypothetical case it might be argued that our vagrant may not know what is in his best interests. To an observer this character may "need treatment" but not recognize his need. The argument now moves from self-serving rationales (e.g., "I want to remove a scandal") to beneficence; (e.g., I wish to help him"); and when those bringing commitment proceedings appear beneficent, the modern court has shown itself to be "all ears." In fact, in a few states the law authorizes involuntary hospitalization under the "need for treatment" rationale (Ennis & Siegel, 1973). That rationale places our hypothetical character in risk of finding himself in the very same place we found him 300 years ago, only now he seems to have been "done in" by benevolence. Instead of banishing Cain or imprisoning him, we now hospitalize him in order to treat him. Instead of punishment, we have *paternalism*.

3

Our hypothetical case stands before us today as he did in the classical age, only now, in this section, it is our conduct that is in question: should we remove him, against his will, for his own good?

The argument against paternalistic interference has been most clearly and forcibly stated by John Stuart Mill, in his essay *On Liberty*. In his words (Mill, 1930):

> The only purpose for which power can rightfully be exercised over any member of a civilized community against his will is to prevent harm to others. . . . His own good, either physical or moral, is not a sufficient warrant. He cannot rightfully be compelled to do or forbear because it will be better for him to do so, because it will make him happier, because, in the opinion of others, to do so would be wise, or even right. These are good reasons for remonstrating with him or reasoning with him, or persuading him, or entreating him, but not for compelling him.

Mill articulated the *harm principle* as the only grounds that justified state coercion: if the individual's actions produce harm to others, the state can justifiably coerce or punish. Mill made it quite clear that neither an offensive moral practice nor a potential personal benefit for the person is sufficient to justify coercion
22   (Beauchamp, 1977).

Avoiding Responsibility
and Assuming It

Following his own principles, Mill would no doubt tell us to leave the poor chap unharmed. Mill might wish to reason with the fellow, perhaps on the topic of assuming and avoiding responsibility; he might urge the fellow to further his education, acquire a job, and elevate his moral conduct; he might even remonstrate, entreat, and plead. Yet he would not compel.

Mill's social philosophy strikes a sympathetic cord with our psychology as well, with many feeling a certain repugnance to the word "paternalism." "To many the word refers to the control of the needs and conduct of others in a heavy-handed, fatherly fashion. But this is not a fair characterization of philosophical and legal uses of the term, and paternalism is by no means a widely discredited practice" (Beauchamp, 1977, p. 10). Beauchamp (1977) tells us that "Recently ethical and legal philosophers have shown a revival of interest in whether paternalistic reasons are ever good reasons for the limitation of individual liberties in the form of coercive laws. A special target has been John Stuart Mill, whose searching criticisms of paternalism in *On Liberty* are now widely regarded as too sweeping and insufficiently guarded." (p. 1).

Several modern social philosophers (Hart, 1963; Dworkin, 1972; Feinberg, 1973) suggest "limits" on Mill's principles, pointing out, on the one hand, that paternalistic laws do exist, but, more importantly, that there might be proper justifications for these paternalistic limits. For example, laws prohibiting a man from selling himself into slavery, bartering himself to a doctor for some form of new and dangerous experiment, or taking morphine purely for the sake of pleasure may be viewed as examples of paternalistic laws (Beauchamp, 1977; Hart, 1963).

Mill's firmly drawn line against coercion has not held historically (Kittrie, 1971), and it has been suggested that "there has been a general decline in the belief that individuals always or even frequently know their own interest best or are capable of free, informed consent" (Beauchamp, 1977, p. 13). Perhaps Mill gives man too much credit, defending too strongly the individual's right to be different and left alone. If we give man less credit, as Hart suggests we are apt to do, then a modern philosopher or psychologist might argue that our Dickensian character does not know his best interest, and therefore the state might properly assume responsibility for him.

THE MEANING OF PATERNALISM
AND ITS ETHICAL DEFENSES

Beauchamp (1977 p. 11) and Dworkin (1972, p. 65), when taken together, provide a fairly precise definition of "paternalism": Paternalism is the coercive interference with a person's liberty of action justified by reasons referring exclusively to the welfare, good, happiness, needs, interests, or values of the person being coerced.

It may be useful to distinguish three types of paternalism (Feinberg, 1973; Beauchamp, 1977):

1. *Legal paternalism:* The justification of state coercion to protect individuals from self-inflicted harm (even if they do not freely consent to the protection).
2. *Extreme paternalism:* The justification of state coercion to benefit individual persons (even if the affected individuals do not regard the coercion as beneficial).
3. *Moral paternalism:*[1] The justification of state coercion to prevent individuals from perform-

---

[1] Beauchamp (1977) points out that others have called this type "legal moralism," but I accept his reasoning for a paternalism label.

ing private immoral acts (even if the affected individuals do not regard the acts as immoral).

Regarding *legal paternalism,* the state may pass laws preventing citizens from injuring themselves (e.g., laws prohibiting suicide), and a policeman may forcibly prevent a man from jumping from a window because "he is sworn to protect life" (Robinson, 1974).

Regarding *extreme paternalism,* Robinson (1974) states as follows:

> This principle was most fully articulated by Plato in *Laws* and *Republic.* According to it, the State must guide the moral development of its citizens, must save them from the corruptions that are intrinsic to the masses. It is based on the belief that the public at large lacks the discipline, motivation, and talent necessary to protect its own interests, even to *learn* its own interests. Arguments for a philosopher-King, for a benign dictator, for the State as suprapublic all rest on this principle. (p. 234)

It also allows the policeman to intervene with the man at the window ledge because he believes the man does not know what is in his own best interests.

Regarding *moral paternalism,* Robinson states (1974), "There are cogent arguments which insist that the notion of civilized society is an empty one unless it is granted that certain moral precepts are common to its members. To this extent, the State may justly prevent actions that ignore or defy moral convention. To remove this principle from that puritanical context for which modern society has such little patience, I offer the torture of animals as an example. . . . The torture of animals involves no harm to human beings; it offends no one if practiced privately. Yet, it is judged to be unconscionable by the public and it is outlawed by the State" (p. 233–4). Similarly, the policeman may intervene with the man at the window ledge because the law judges suicide to be immoral.

Applying these three types of paternalism to our hypothetical character, we can justify his forcible removal from his sidewalk spot because (a) he is likely to harm himself by his actions (e.g., the absence of socks during cold weather may be "liberally" construed as leading, in likelihood, to illness, or suicide by degree), and thus legal paternalism could be invoked; (b) he does not know what is in his own best interests (extreme paternalism); and (c) that to "hang out" is a fall from the proper moral order of things, as it was in the classical age (Foucault, 1973), and hence is action that justifies intervention (moral paternalism).

Our character, even with his tattered copy of Constitution, may not be able to weather this philosophical downpour. In being pried loose from Mill's protective umbrella—in the name of his own "welfare, good, happiness, needs, interests, or values"—he is about to be taken to a place of safety and shelter to dry out from the storm. He is going to a state psychiatric hospital.

If he cries out to the heavens, to his street-corner audience, or to his assailants, "I'm being railroaded!" "Let me go!" "I'm a free man!," does he not deserve a reply? But what reply?

Beauchamp (1977), who has surveyed the proposed justifications for coercion, cites four grounds:

(i) There exist reasonable grounds for believing that the individual(s) affected either (a) do not know what is in their best interest, yet what is best in their own interest can be ascertained... (b) do know what is in their best interest, yet are in some circumstances insufficiently motivated to pursue that interest unless legally required to do so....
(ii) A "wider range of freedom for the individual in question" is achieved by some paternalistic interference....
(iii) An extreme risk which is manifestly unreasonable "in respect to its objectively assessable components" can be avoided by paternalistic interference....
(iv) Decisions "which are far-reaching, potentially dangerous and irreversible" and which pertain exclusively to "goods" such as health (analogous to education for children) can be controlled by paternalistic interference so that disasters or intrinsic evils do not befall citizens—provided that no value in the form of a competing reason (not an irrational one) is mentioned by the individual" (pp. 17-18)

Let us take a closer look at each of these reasons, and gauge its implications for our sidewalk superintendent. It might be argued at his commitment hearing that he does not know what is in his own best interest. Yet who is doing the arguing? His family? Or the state? Can they, or we, really "ascertain" what is *his* best interest? Does *our* answer, in the last analysis, become no more than *our own projection*—a paternalistic projection—which denies to him, but not to us, "personal responsibility" (Szasz, 1970)? In order to argue on this ground for coercion, first we must show that he does not know. Second, we would have to ascertain whether this lack of knowing results from a lack of information, a deficiency in education, inadequate reflection, or internal confusion. A lack of information, deficiency in education, or inadequate reflection can be corrected without the heavy hand of coercion. So it is only in the last case, the case of not knowing because of internal confusion — being mentally ill — that the argument takes on force.

Looking at part (b) of (i), where the best interest is known but not followed, can we hospitalize someone against his will to treat him (psychologically, chemically, or surgically), even though he acknowledges that the treatment may help, but steadfastly maintains his right to refuse? This hypothetical situation can be applied to the late Supreme Court Justice, Robert Jackson:

> Robert Jackson was a Justice on the United States Supreme Court. He developed a serious heart condition and was warned by his doctors that unless he retired from the court and led a very restricted life, he would probably die within a few months. Justice Jackson decided to stay on the Court anyway, and died a few months later of a heart attack. He had the right to make such a choice. Similarly, a patient in a general hospital may refuse to undergo an operation even if his life depends upon it. He has the absolute right, if he is conscious, to make the choice between surgery and almost certain death. And if that right is violated, he has good grounds to sue the doctor for assault and battery. (From Ennis J, Siegel L: The Rights of Mental Patients. Copyright 1973 by the American Civil Liberties Union Inc. Reprinted by permission of Avon Books, New York.)

What if, however, as in the above example pertaining to (i)(a), the argument is made that the person in question is mentally ill? Ennis and Siegel answer:

> For mental patients, the situation is just the opposite. In many states, the mental patient's consent is not required either for emergency or *nonemergency surgery*.[2] Instead, the superintendent, the hospital board, or a relative (even if he committed the patient in the first place) may make that very important decision. Why is it that Justice Jackson could refuse to retire and a general patient could refuse emergency surgery, but a mental patient may not refuse even nonemergency surgery? The answer is that it is generally believed that mental patients are not competent to give or withhold rational consent." (p. 69)

So the argument (b) of (i), like part (a), returns to the question and issue of mental illness as the disqualifier of our right to refuse.

Justification (ii) is that a wider range of freedom could be achieved by some paternalistic interference. Let us see how it can be applied to our running example. Let me make a nineteenth century assertion coupled with a twentieth century technique:

---

[2] Nonemergency surgery is surgery not necessary to save the patient's life.

what if it is now argued that our sidewalk superintendent suffers from a defect in the moral center of his brain, and that psychosurgery (i.e., a technique whereby a microelectrode is appropriately placed in a particular brain section and DC current is applied with the intent of destroying those cells that contact the wire) would destroy the vagrant cells producing the vagrant behavior, thus freeing the person from his illness and allowing him "a wider range of freedom." Can it be morally done? Even over his protests? The argument in (ii) seems to reduce, as it did in (i)(a) and (i)(b), to the question of mental illness. We now add to our ethical question empirical questions of brain localized functions; but the cutting edge of the question is still mental illness. People in their "right mind" can refuse psychosurgery, neurosurgery, or any type of surgery, even if it may widen their freedom. However, once it has been argued and decided that the person is of "wrong mind," that right to refuse is undermined.

Criterion (iii) is troubled on several accounts. Using potential violence, be it suicide or homicide, as an example, how do we know when the "extreme-risk" point has been reached, and how do we judge "objectively assessable components"? Both terms are riddled with inexactness, and hence easily fall prey to differing subjective assessments. We know, for example, that our predictions of dangerous acts are notoriously poor, and we usually tended to overjudge dangerousness by a considerable degree (Rappaport, 1977). A man at home with a gun may be seen as an example of our constitutional right to bear arms; but assert that he is mentally ill and see how quickly our assessment changes. Criterion (iii), like (ii), (i)(a), and (i)(b) before it, reduces to the issue of right or wrong mind.

Criterion (iv) is no different. Take the hypothetical case of a 22-year-old promiscuous girl, who has been in and out of various hospitals, therapies, and concubinage, and, as a result of the latter, has an illegitimate child. Her parents support the child. She continues to act out sexually and refuses sterilization. Can she be sterilized over her strenuous objections? Here is the argument that sterilization, or the lack of it, has "far-reaching, potentially dangerous, and irreversible" consequences for health, and that it ought to be left to the state, rather than the individual to decide. The case of *Buck* v. *Bell*[3] touched on just this question (Kittrie, 1971):

> In 1927, however, Justice Holmes, speaking for the United States Supreme Court in *Buck* v. *Bell*, laid these due process objections to

---

[3] 274 U. S. 200 (1927).

rest and upheld sterilization as falling within the permissible constitutional dimensions. Carrie Buck was committed to a Virginia mental institution as mentally deficient. Both her mother and her own illegitimate daughter were similarly feebleminded. Under the state's procedure for effecting sterilization, it was determined that the best interest of the patient and society would be served if Miss Buck was infertile. The Supreme Court addressed itself to the substantive issue of whether the state had the power to order the sterilization of an individual for eugenic purposes. The state's interest in the maintenance of the quality of the species, Holmes held, was superior to any individual's power of procreation. . . . The often quoted rationale is summarized by Justice Holmes:

We have seen more than once that the public welfare may call upon the best citizens for their lives. It would be strange if it could not call upon those who already sap the strength of the State for these lesser sacrifices, often not felt to be such by those concerned, in order to prevent our being swamped with incompetence. It is better for all the world, if instead of waiting to execute degenerate offspring for crime, or to let them starve for their imbecility, society can prevent those who are manifestly unfit from continuing their kind. The principle that sustains compulsory vaccination is broad enough to cover cutting the fallopian tubes. . . . Three generations of imbeciles are enough. (pp. 318–319)

Holmes and the Court made a decision then that, in all probability, they would reverse today. Many of the genetic assumptions that were accepted at that time have since been discredited. For example, the odds of retarded individuals having retarded offspring are small; secondly, 80–90 percent of the retarded are born to normal individuals. Thus, had Holmes and the rest of the Court had at their disposal knowledge that is now "current," it is likely that the decision would have been quite different. Yet the point is that the courts have leaned and still do lean heavily on the "current" psychological thinking of the age, even when that psychological foundation is infirm.

Buck presented the case of a mentally retarded woman. What would have happened if there were another case where it was asserted that the female was mentally ill? And if it were shown that she came from a troubled family, and that her child was showing "signs" of trouble, would it have been argued analogously that "three generations of mental illness are enough"?

The common denominator and deciding factor in these criteria boils down to our "current" beliefs regarding mental illness. Before exploring the current status of mental illness, let us turn back to its historical status and the beginning practice of paternalism.

PATERNALISM IN HISTORY

The practice of paternalism seems traceable to a concept rooted in common law, that the king has a benevolent role to play as part of his sovereignty, since he is "the guardian of his people" (Kittrie, 1971). *Parens patriae* became the term to designate the king's fatherly role in raising his subjects. According to early documents of the English kings, the *parens patriae* power was limited by tradition—a tradition whereby local feudal lords or ecclesiastics cared for the ill and disabled. With this arrangement, the king could ignore, for the most part, his less fortunate subjects. However, some changes in the limited use of this power were already evident in the eleventh century enactments of King Aethelred II, nicknamed "the Unready," who extended his protection to any wise man or stranger whose orders, goods, or life were endangered. To these subjects, the king was saying, "I will act as your kinsman and protector, if you have none." The chief beneficiaries of this revised policy were not the wise men but the incompetent subjects.

In the fourteenth century, King Edward II claimed a proprietary interest in the insane. A *parens patriae* intervention prevented heirs and feudal lords from confiscating the insane man's assets, while asserting the Crown's right to them. Regal confiscation was backed by the Church so that the Church could be repaid for its philanthropy.

From these beginning steps, the *parens patriae* role has been asserted with a growing frequency that has continued to the present, and usually (J.S. Mill notwithstanding) it has been backed by public approval. One area where this can be clearly seen is in the historical trend and process of "divestment," whereby "noncriminal controls and procedures have usurped areas previously claimed by criminal law" (p. 32). For example, in the fourteenth century, England exempted insane murderers from criminal responsibility. It was held, by both beneficent father and budding social scientist (whose flowering and positivist growth was still several centuries away), that to punish the insane was ineffective as a deterrent, since hanging a lunatic taught no lesson to a sane man. What began to make more sense in these cases was to temper the control measures to fit the offender rather than the crime.

Mercy, rather than *severity,* was urged, and treatment, rather than punishment, was tried.

It is clear that the Crown was *not* entirely clear and consistent on this matter of divestment, as witnessed by the behavior of Queen Victoria in the famous trial and acquittal of Daniel M'Naghten[4]:

> The M'Naghten Rules are to be found, as we have said, in eight English Reports, Reprint, at p. 722 et seq. (1843), and were engendered by the excitement and fear which grew out of the acquittal of Daniel M'Naghten who had attempted to assassinate Sir Robert Peel, Prime Minister of England, but who instead shot Peel's private secretary, Drummond, because M'Naghten had mistaken Drummond for Peel. The offense against Drummond followed a series of attempted assassinations of members of the English Royal House, including Queen Victoria herself, and attacks on the Queen's ministers. When M'Naghten was acquitted at his trial[5], public indignation, led by the Queen, ran so high that the judges of England were called before the House of Lords to explain their conduct. A series of questions were propounded to them. Their answers, really an advisory opinion which (sic.) delivered by Lord Chief Justice Tindal for all fifteen judges, save Mr. Justice Maule, constitute what are now known as the M'Naghten Rules. These Rules have fastened themselves on the law of England and on the law of almost all of the States and on all of the federal courts save one. (pp. 763–764)

Although the murder in high places by insane minds incensed Queen Victoria, it did not stop the process of divestment and its *parens patriae* rationale. By the late nineteenth century, juvenile offenders were exempted from traditional criminal proceedings, and today, psychopaths, hysterics, drug addicts, and chronic alcoholics have joined the ranks of the schizophrenics and psychotics as divestment groups, "removed from the jurisdiction of the criminal law" (Kittrie, 1971, p. 33). But more on that later.

For now, it is important to note the *trend* and its supporting assertions: that the insane did not have *mens rea* ("evil mind" or awareness of wrongdoing); that the insane did not have free will; that punishment of them was inappropriate, ineffective, and "cruel and unusual"; and that humanism and mercy, with dictate treatment, should replace the harsh controls and severity of retributive punishment that marked an earlier age.

Beneficence costs, however, and the price is personal respon-

---

[4] *United States* v. *Currens,* 290 F 2d 751 (1961).

[5] *Regina* v. *M'Naghten,* 4 State Trials, N.S. 923 (1843).

sibility. To be freed of criminal responsibility, the case was made that the person lacked personal responsibility: he was not a moral agent, but sick, or as a child. Whether or not he never had responsibility in the first place, or just avoided exercising it, the parenting state would assume that responsibility and prescribe treatment. The "patient" was about to be wrapped in a therapeutic blanket.

Would the State, however, be wrapped in its own self-deception? Would the State be tricked by its apparent beneficence, only to hide its controlling intent? Was *parens patriae* a soothing of our egalitarian conscience, which permitted us to place these "unfortunates" in a "controlled," therapeutic environment while maintaining our night's sleep? The State, for the most part, neither examined nor answered these questions. In the words of Szasz (1970), "The 'benevolent' despot, whether political or psychiatric, does not like to have his benevolence questioned" (p. 39).

Yet it is Szasz who questions and answers, and who sees in the *parens patriae* benevolence a counterviolence that is moral and political in nature. He writes:

> My approach to psychiatry as essentially a moral and political enterprise led me to reappraise numerous situations in which this perspective appeared most promising of new insights — such as education, law, the control of conception and of drug abuse, politics, and, of course, psychiatry itself. In each instance, I tried to show that, on the one hand, by seeking relief from the burden of his moral responsibilities, man mystifies and technicizes his problems in living, and that, on the other hand, the demand for "help" thus generated is now met by a behavioral technology ready and willing to free man of his moral burdens by treating him as a sick patient. . . . Indeed, when the justificatory rhetoric with which the oppressor conceals and misrepresents his true aims and methods is most effective . . . the oppressor succeeds not only in subduing his victim but also in robbing him of a vocabulary for articulating his victimization, thus making him a captive deprived of all means of escape. (pp. 3–5)

Paternalism has grown, but not without pangs of conscience and mental anguish in those supposed to be free of that sort of thing. Its motivation, rooted in humanism and equated with an enlightened consciousness, casts a dark shadow that taints its practices and questions its intent. In its light and dark forms, paternalism presents us with paradox.

THE SHIP OF FOOLS

In 1494, two years after Columbus' sea voyage to the new world, Sebastian Brant (Zeydel, 1944) wrote a book, *Das Narrenschiff* (the ship of fools) which reflected the practices of his day; the idea of the ship, its cargo, and its purpose, had meaning rooted in a much older world. In the late fifteenth century, men would only reenact those earlier rites of exclusion, purification, and renewal, whereby men of reason would rid themselves of unreason, or at least tell themselves they did.

Here are some of Brant's words on the subject:

A PROLOGUE TO THE SHIP OF FOOLS
For profit and salutary instruction, admonition and pursuit of wisdom, reason and good manners: also for contempt and punishment of folly, blindness, error, and stupidity of all stations and kinds of men: with special zeal, earnestness, and labor compiled at Basel by Sebastian Brant, doctor in both laws.

All lands in Holy Writ abound
And works to save the soul are found,
The Bible, Holy Fathers' lore
And other such in goodly store,
So many that I feel surprise
To find men growing not more wise
But holding writ and lore in spite.
The whole world lives in darksome night,
In blinded sinfulness persisting,
While every street sees fools existing
Who know but folly, to their shame,
Yet will not own to folly's name.
Hence I have pondered how a ship
Of fools I'd suitably equip—
A galley, brig, bark, skiff, or float,
A carack, scow, dredge, racing-boat,
A sled, cart, barrow, carryall—

One vessel would be far too small
To carry all the fools I know.
Forgive me what I say, I would
Not wish to injure their good name,
I'd stress the bad ones' evil fame,
Full scores of whom deserve a trip
Aboard our crowded idiot's ship.

With caution everyone should look
To see if he's in this my book,
And who thinks not will say that he
Of wand and fool's cap may be free.
Who thinks that he is not affected
To wise men's doors be he directed,
There let him wait until mayhap
From Frankfurt I can fetch a cap.

As mentioned above, this rite is not new. Sir James George
Frazer, in his classic, *The Golden Bough* (1963), traces the ancient rites of transferring evil to objects, and then to animals (the
scapegoat), and then to men; what followed this transference of
evil was their periodic, public expulsion. He cites one practice in
the southern district of the island of Ceram where a little ship or
boat is readied, laden with rice, tobacco, eggs, etc., and a man

> Calls out in a very loud voice, "O all ye sicknesses, ye smallpoxes,
> agues, measles, etc., who have visited us so long and wasted us so
> sorely, but who now cease to plague us, we have made ready this
> ship for you, and we have furnished you with provender sufficient
> for the voyage. Ye shall have no lack of food nor of betel-leaves nor
> of areca nuts nor ot tobacco. Depart, and sail away from us directly;
> never come near us again; but go to a land which is far from here.
> Let all the tides and winds waft you speedily thither, and so convey
> you thither that for the time to come we may live sound and well,
> and that we may never see the sun rise on you again." (p. 653)

It was only a short step to add *man* to the cargo list. Frazer
cites the practices of the Banyoro, where the scapegoat is "either
a man and a boy or a woman and her child, chosen because of
some mark or bodily defect, which the gods had noted and by
which the victims were to be recognized" (p. 655). Now, returning
to the fifteenth century, the cargo is the *fool*.

Some clarification is in order. It must be made clear exactly
who the fool is, what "marks" him, and what he represents (Foucault, 1973). First, he is not the Shakespearean fool—the jester
who quips and somersaults between Acts I and II; and he is not
the dullard, lacking sense or IQ points. The image of folly in the
Renaissance was linked to Unreason, Evil, the Fall from morality, and Death. He is reason distorted, the truth blinded. He is
linked with wickedness, lewdness, and perverse morality. He has
linked himself with darkness, compacted with Satan, and em-
blematized the Antichrist. The fool's grin is likened to the grin of
the skeleton, the grin of death; for the fool portends death, since
his head is half empty already. The face of the fool is mirrored in

Albrecht Durer's woodcuts, in the images of the Apocalypse Horsemen; he is the beast, our monstrous subterranean forms that haunt our nightmares. He now stalks Europe.

Carl Jung, another doctor from Basel, might smile and nod knowingly hearing this description. He would not miss man's *shadow,* embodied in the particular form of the fool and projected from the unconscious to mirror and complete man's *persona*: "Reason, meet Unreason." Did Sebastian Brant miss his projection?

It is clear that many missed it. We know from Brant's biography that he was deeply disturbed by the corruption he saw in the Church a half century before Luther. He saw open sensuality inside the church; he saw prostitutes openly solicit in the church aisles, lovers getting up and embracing, and he heard sermons from the pulpit that were immodest, if not licentious. Brant was not advocating reformation, but repentence: he was looking for a Church, societal, and personal cleansing – the rites of exclusion, purification, and renewal. He was the perfect author of a book that perfectly captured his age. We know. The book sold.

One book that did not sell was Erasmus' *Moriae Encomium, In Praise of Folly,* which presented a different view of folly and its relation to reason. Erasmus saw man as both reason and folly, conscious and unconscious, persona and shadow – the union of opposites. He could not deny *our* madness; it would be madness to deny it – to *project* it – onto someone else. Erasmus' view, however, was psychologically more threatening than Brant's, and it was denied by the public of his day. The counter-reformation helped to revive it and bring it into the private libraries and thoughts of seventeenth century Frenchmen, but in its day it bombed at the box office.

There was a third view, expressed most vividly by Hieronymus Bosch in his paintings *The Ship of Fools* and *The Cure of Folly.* Bosch's visionary view caught the conflict and its surrealistic quality. The "cure" for folly, administered by a doctor with a dunce cap-like funnel on his head and attended by a monk and a nun, the latter with a book balanced on her head, was but another form of madness. The foolishness of medicine teamed up with religious folly. The fate of Bosch, and this could be said of other visionaries, was that he painted for a blind audience. In that age, the dominant view of madness was not Bosch's, but Brant's.

So they rounded up the mad and shipped them out on an odyssey to who knows where. Perhaps they were destined to be destroyed on their death boat – to be swallowed up by the sea as their reason had been swallowed up by madness. Perhaps this was a fool's sea voyage, to be wandering endlessly, like the fool's life, undertaken without rudder and compass; this was a directionless journey, mirroring a wasted, directionless life. Their rescue could come only from God.

Their fate, drowning or rescue, was in God's hands. The irony became complete: God, the one who was rejected in the error-filled life of the fool, becomes his sole redeemer.

Whether this sea story of a boat and its cargo made it to a fool's utopia, to some shrine or city that welcomed these pilgrims and offered them sanctuary, is a story without an ending. It cannot be written by anyone who has stayed on land. Men of Reason can only look at their own behavior and story, and see in it the confirmation of the Reason–Madness nexus; Madness was to be split from Reason within the psyche and the community; it seems Reason needed it that way. The exclusion of Madness purified Reason.

LETTRES DE CACHET

To men like Erasmus, Bosch, and Jung, all of whom embraced both Reason and Folly, the exclusion of darkness by the light of consciousness must seem like madness itself, destined to fail. And fail it did. What was next to be tried historically, was inclusion – the confinement of madness – by reason of *lettres de cachet*.

> By a strange act of force, the classical age was to reduce to silence the madness whose voices the Renaissance had just liberated, but whose violence it had already tamed.
>
> It is common knowledge that the seventeenth century created enormous houses of confinement; it is less commonly known that more than one out of every hundred inhabitants of the city of Paris found themselves confined there, within several months. It is common knowledge that absolute power made use of *lettres de cachet* and arbitrary measures of imprisonment; what is less familiar is the judicial conscience that could inspire such practices. (Foucault, 1973, p. 38)

From exclusion aboard boats to confinement within the Hôpital Général, the *forms* of paternalism were changing as the Renaissance was giving way to the classical age. By royal decree (1656), the Hôpital Général was founded in Paris. The German counterpart was called *Zuchthaus;* the English, *house of correction.* And by another Royal decree, this time in the form of a letter, the recipient gained kingly contact, only to lose his freedom. "For the first time, purely negative measures of exclusion were replaced by a measure of confinement; the unemployed person was no longer driven away or punished; he was taken in charge, at the expense of the nation but at the cost of his individual liberty. Between him and society, an implicit system of obligation was established: he had the right to be fed, but he must accept the physical and moral constraint of confinement." (Foucault, 1973, p. 48)

If we examine more closely this change in paternalistic tactic, this new approach of dealing with madness, we see a confusion of motives that mixes severity with mercy and confounds treatment with punishment. The madman's "best interests" may have been cited, but the practice of confinement belies beneficence. Peeking into these not-so-hidden motives reveals "a moral institution responsible for punishing, for correcting a certain moral abeyence which does not merit the tribunal of men, but cannot be corrected by the severity of penance alone. The Hôpital Général has an ethical status. It is this moral charge which invests its director, and they are granted every judicial apparatus and means of repression: 'They have power of authority, of direction, of administration, of commerce, of police, of jurisdiction, of correction and punishment'; and to accomplish this task 'stakes, irons, prisons, and dungeons' are put at their disposal" (p. 59).

Hearing all of these quotes, our hypothetical Dickensian character begins to shudder and gets that "paranoid" feeling that his liberty is in jeopardy. The *lettres de cachet,* and their "deliverers," are on their way. The mendicants, beggars, and vagabonds are rounded up. The squanderers, madmen, and blasphemers, the young and the old, all get their letters. "Hôpital" may sound like "hospital," but these houses of confinement were not medical establishments. "It is rather a sort of semijudicial structure, an administrative entity which, along with the already constituted powers, and outside of the courts, decides, judges, and executes" (p. 40).

They executed a "punishment–treatment" plan of *work.* The idle were given work – they were forced to work – as punishment and penance for their Fall. There were more sinister motives too. Confinement of the poor sequestered a potentially dangerous section of the population who might revolt against the established order; confinement of well placed persons also occurred; with both, a preventive, political measure could be hidden in the alleged treatment through confinement. Economic exploitation also figured into the practice. Confined bodies were cheap labor; if they could be utilized, a profit might be turned. In Germany each *Zuchthaus* had its specialty: "Spinning was paramount in Bremen, Brunswick, Munich, Breslan, Berlin; weaving in Hanover.

The men shredded wood in Bremen and Hamburg. In Nuremberg they polished optical glass; at Mainz the principal labor was the milling of flour" (pp. 51–52).

They did not turn a profit, however. It failed economically as it failed therapeutically, because it was not therapy—in the volitional, contractual sense of therapy as we know it today. The madman, along with the rest of the idlers, was being punished, excluded, and confined in former leprosariums that were quickly being renamed "hôpitaux"; the change of name and treatment population (from leprosarium to hopital, and from leper to madman) could neither hide a consistent pattern of moral and ethical judgment and punishment, nor veil in therapeutic euphemisms its deeper intent.

> Madness was thus torn from that imaginary freedom which still allowed it to flourish on the Renaissance horizon. Not so long ago, it had floundered about in broad daylight: in *King Lear,* in *Don Quixote.* But in less than a half-century, it had been sequestered and, in the fortress of confinement, bound to reason, to the rules of morality and to their monotonous nights (Foucault, 1973, p. 64).

The state's practice of using *lettres de cachet* continues, although the name has changed. Recently, through accounts of Soviet immigrants and dissidents, the Soviet practice of using "psychiatric terror" to suppress dissent and promote confinement has been revealed (Bloch & Reddaway, 1977; Solzhenitsyn, 1974). In one account (Szasz, 1970, p. 29), a Jewish poet, Iosif Brodsky, was brought to trial for "pursuing a parasitic way of life," for example, poetry, which was not considered "productive" or "socially useful labor." Brodsky was ordered to undergo an official psychiatric examination to determine whether he was "laboring" under some form of psychological disorder which was, in turn, causing him to labor unproductively.

So the state's use of letters to intern psychiatrically someone who may threaten the state by his actions or views continues, as does the paternalistic cover up. Politics and psychology continue to mix, but the taste is sour, and the therapy, spoiled.

Returning to the classical age for a moment, the use of *lettres* quickly passed from king to parent to spouse to almost anyone who adopted or feigned "paternalistic" interest. If a citizen was concerned with the mental health of another, he could seek internment in a madhouse by filing a *lettre*—"due reason, inquiry, and authority" would come later—if at all.

The "perversion" of this spread of paternalism is seen most clearly in the complaint of Daniel Defoe (1661–1731), a journalist and novelist, who was also an early critic of psychiatric confinement (Szasz, 1973):

This leads me to exclaim against the vile Practice now so much in vogue among the better Sort, as they are called, but the worst sort in fact, namely, the sending their Wives to Mad-Houses at every Whim or Dislike, that they may be more secure and undisturb'd in their Debaucheries: Which wicked Custom is got to such a Head, that the number of private Mad-Houses in and about London, are considerably increased within these few Years. This is the height of Barbarity and Injustice in a Christian Country, it is a clandestine Inquisition, nay worse. How many Ladies and Gentlewomen are hurried away to these Houses, which ought to be suppress'd, or at least subject to daily Examination, as hereafter shall be proposed? How many, I say, of Beauty, Vertue, and Fortune, are suddenly torn from their dear innocent Babes, from the Arms of an unworthy Man, who they love (perhaps too well) and who in Return for that Love, nay probably an ample Fortune, and a lovely Offspring besides; grows weary of the pure Streams of chaste Love, and thirsting for the Puddles of lawless Lust, buries his vertuous Wife alive, that he may have the greater Freedom with his Mistresses?

If they are not mad when they go into these cursed Houses, they are soon made so by the barbarous Usage they there suffer, and any Woman of spirit who has the least Love for her Husband, or Concern for her family, cannot sit down tamely under a Confinement and Separation the most unaccountable and unreasonable. Is it not enough to make any one mad to be suddenly clap'd up, stripp'd, whipp'd, ill fed, and worse us'd? To have no Reason assign'd for such Treatment, no Crime alledg'd, or accusers to confront? And what is worse, no Soul to appear to but merciless Creatures, who answer but in Laughter, Surliness, Contradiction, and too often Stripes? All conveniences for Writing are denied, no Messenger to be had to carry a Letter to any Relation or Friend; and if this tyrannical Inquisition, join'd with the reasonable Reflections, a woman of any common Understanding must necessarily make, be not sufficient to drive any Soul stark staring mad, though before they were never so much in their right Senses, I have no more to say....

How many are yet to be sacrificed, unless a speedy Stop be put to this most accursed Practice I tremble to think; our Legislature cannot take this Cause too soon in hand: This surely cannot be below their Notice, and twill be an easy matter at once to suppress all these pretended Mad-Houses. Indulge, gentle Reader, for once the doing of an old Man, and give him leave to lay down his little System without arraigning him of Arrogance or Ambition to be a Law-giver. In my humble Opinion all private Mad-Houses should be suppress'd at once, and it should be no less than Felony to confine any Person under pretence of Madness without due Authority. For the cure of those who are really Lunatick, licens'd Mad-Houses should be constituted in convenient Parts of the Town, which Houses should be subject to proper Visitation and Inspection, nor should any Person be sent to a Mad-House without due Reason, Inquiry and Authority. (pp. 7–9)

"DUE REASON, INQUIRY, AND AUTHORITY"—THE PROCESS OF CONFINEMENT

On both sides of the Atlantic concern was voiced for *procedural* requirements and safeguards to replace the loose, informal, and often cavalier manner by which commitment had been instigated in past ages. While several states (e.g., Massachusetts, New Hampshire, Connecticut) had some form of safeguards by the mid-nineteenth century, many more did not. One crusader for tighter commitment laws in the United States in the 1860s was Mrs. Packard, an expatient; she attempted to "arouse public concern in order to make 'railroading' to lunatic asylums impossible" (Kittrie, 1971, p. 65). Szasz (1970, p. 117) provides some details of the Packard case: for one, it seems she was "incarcerated for disagreeing with her minister-husband": for another, "the commitment laws of the State of Illinois explicitly proclaimed that '... married women... may be interred or detained in the hospital at the request of the husband of the woman or the guardian. ..; without the evidence of insanity required in other cases.'" It would appear that Mrs. Packard had a point.

As a result of her exposés, many formal guarantees of due process, such as a hearing and a jury trial, were introduced. The procedural safeguards had at least three advantages: they protected patients against "railroading" where the motivations of the one instituting commitment were frivolous, arbitrary, or, as Defoe said, "at every Whim or Dislike"; they protected the institutional officials against suits claiming malfeasance and wrongful detention; and they protected the institution from being overrun by paupers and vagabonds who were willing to be admitted to gain institutional benefits such as food and shelter.

Today each state has its own laws governing involuntary admissions. In general these laws differ significantly from state to state, and they differ on substantive and procedural grounds. 'Substantive" grounds concern the criteria states adopt to sanction involuntary admissions, such as "mentally ill," or "dangerous," or "dangerous to self or others," or "needs treatment." Different states have different criteria, and even where the same criteria exist, they may have different operational definitions for these terms (i.e., what is "mentally ill" or "dangerous" in one state may not be in another). "Procedural" grounds, which again differ widely from state to state, concern the specific steps of the commitment process. Can lay citizens institute commitment procedures, or must the commitment be medically sanctioned or judicially issued? These questions are answered differently in different states. So are questions concerning the right to notice; the right to have counsel present; guarantees against self-incrimination; the opportunity to be heard; and the rights to cross-examine, to free expert witnesses if one cannot afford them, to trial by one's peers, and to proof beyond a reasonable doubt (Ennis & Siegel, 1973, Kittrie, 1971).

In this section the commitment process will be reviewed with a look toward (a) what steps are taken; (b) what rationales are offered; and (c) what part the mental health professional, family, lawyer, patient, court, and community play in this drama.

THE PERCEPTION OF A PROBLEM WORTHY
OF HOSPITALIZATION

To begin with, the prospective patient usually has to engage in some behavior that is *troubling to others* before steps to hospitalize are undertaken. Smith, Pumphrey, and Hall (1973) have reviewed the decisive incidents—the "last straw" as they call them —which led family, neighbors, or police to decide that this person should no longer remain in the community or family, and that hospitalization was essential. They studied, in retrospective fashion, 100 schizophrenic patients and their 100 last straws. They divided the incidents into three broad categories: (a) behavior that was seen as actually or potentially harmful to the patient or others (e.g., suicidal threats or attempts, threatening to hit a family member, destruction of property); (b) socially unacceptable behavior (e.g., being nude in a public park, shouting, refusing to talk, irrational talk, using obscene words, inexplicable behavior, wandering, eating a raw chicken); and (c) behaviors indicating mental illness and requiring treatment (e.g., thoughts of losing one's mind, having hallucinations or delusions, being very confused).

We know that people (and communities) differ in their judgments and tolerance of deviancy (Finkel, 1976; Miller, 1967; Yarrow, Schwartz, Murphy, & Deasy, 1973); thus the greater the tolerance of deviancy, the less likely it will be that someone (a family member, for instance) will reach the conclusion that hospitalization is in order. People differ in their judgments of what is dangerous, what is socially unacceptable, and whether treatment is required. Yet if someone reaches that individual judgment, he may take action to hospitalize. Bittner (1973) studied the police practices of a large West Coast city as they related to emergency apprehension of mentally ill persons. Bittner notes the legal facts: officers have statutory authorization to take steps to initiate confinement in a psychiatric hospital if, as a result of their own observations, they reach the judgment that a person is mentally ill and is likely to injure himself or others. Bittner also notes the empirical facts: that police officers are very hesitant to invoke this law because they recognize a lack of competence in matters pertaining to psychopathology. As a result they seem to be very cautious in judging a problem "a psychiatric hospitalization" case. Thus a person would have to be more than just "troublesome"; usually a danger to life, physical health, or property would have to be judged as imminent.

Comparing Bittner's findings with police officers to Smith, Pumphrey, and Hall's (1973) findings regarding "last straws," a clear difference emerges: for Smith and his associates, 47% of the last straws were not dangerous acts (e.g., socially unacceptable behaviors or illnesses judged as requiring treatment). A tentative conclusion might be that family and community members are quicker to reach the psychiatric hospitalization decision than the police. Perhaps their apprehensions are greater, or their patience less; or perhaps they do not see alternatives to hospitalization.

Bittner points out that for the police, the decision to hospitalize "is determined largely by the absence of other alternatives" (p. 48). The police can try (a) to persuade the person to go to a hospital voluntarily, (b) to restore control such that the potential disturbance is less likely, (c) to locate caretakers for the prospective patient, or (d) to give direct psychiatric first aid. If these alternatives fail, involuntary hospitalization is likely. Family members may be in a different boat: they have to live with the troubling behavior and their troubled kin; they may not have the necessary impartiality to convince their kin to seek voluntary hospitalization; they may not have the requisite force to restore control; being the current caretakers, they may see no other alternative care giver other than the mental hospital; and the likelihood is that they have tried giving psychiatric first aid and failed.

Alternatives that the police see and have, relatives may not have or see.

Then there is the "personal stake": this may translate into "we have to save the rest of this family, so he has to go." In an article by Miller and Schwartz (1973) regarding county lunacy commission hearings, they summarize the role of the relatives in the following quote:

> Relatives were also under great strain by virtue of their appearance in the role of the complainant. Their reactions ranged from great shame to profound relief. To interpret these observations as showing that these relatives were engaged in "railroading" their unwanted family member into the mental hospital is to distort reality. The strain of breaking ties of loyalty and of facing up to the public ordeal of commitment was greater indeed. Apparently the complainants took on this role with great distaste and, generally, only after they had experienced long periods of discomfort and dismay. They felt they were in a trap and, for them, the mental hospital seemed to be the only way out. (pp. 132–133)

Now there are two main ways of proceeding: emergency hospitalization and nonemergency hospitalization. (I am assuming in this discussion that voluntary hospitalization has been suggested, and refused.) Emergency hospitalization is supposed to be used only in exceptional cases, since it gives prospective patients fewer rights and safeguards than nonemergency procedures. Exceptional cases are usually those in which the prospective patient would be "imminently dangerous" either to himself or others. Yet, as Ennis and Siegel (1973) point out:

> The first thing to know about "emergency" hospitalization is that it is a misnomer. Emergency hospitalization procedures give the prospective patient many fewer rights and safeguards than he would receive under the *non*emergency procedures, so the "emergency" procedure is supposed to be used only in exceptional cases. In fact, the so-called emergency procedure is, in almost every state, the *standard* procedure and almost everyone is hospitalized, initially, under the emergency procedure, where there is a true emergency or not. In New York City, for example, about 99% of all involuntary patients are hospitalized, initially, under the emergency procedure. (p. 17)

The prospective patient has to be brought to the hospital; this involves an infringement of personal liberty, such as a husband tossing his wife into the back seat of a car and driving her, against her will, to the hospital. Is this "arrest" legal? Ennis and Siegel tell us that this question is not answered by the laws of most states. Lay commitment, where the unsworn allegation by some citizen that a prospective patient is mentally ill and danger-ous, has been sanctioned by some states, although the trend has been, of recent years, to change state laws and eliminate lay commitment. So if someone reaches the conclusion that person A needs hospitalization, he may need either (a) a certificate signed by one or more doctors who have personally examined the pros-pective patient and found him both mentally ill and dangerous to self or others (medical commitment) or (b) a court order (judicial commitment). The latter is not necessarily "håving your day in court," since judges can issue commitment orders without having seen or heard the prospective patient; and the former is not neces-sarily having your mental health examined impartially, since the doctors may be hired by the family member initiating commit-ment.

These, in general, are the varied emergency hospitalization procedures. The underlying rationale, analogous to Mill's *harm principle,* is the immediate protection of the population from a potentially dangerous situation.

OUR BELIEFS AND JUDGMENTS OF DANGEROUSNESS

In our rush to protect, however, might we be too hasty with law and liberty, and in error in our judgment? Regarding the latter point — our judgment of potentially dangerous situations — how accurate are we in predicting dangerousness? Ennis and Siegel (1973) reach an emphatic conclusion: "Perhaps the most serious problem with the danger standard is that psychiatrists . . . know almost nothing about dangerousness. Psychiatrists may or may not be able to tell us whether a prospective patient is mentally ill . . . but they simply cannot tell us whether he is dangerous or will be in the future. That is a strong statement but it is true. In fact, psychiatrists are even *less* accurate in predicting dangerous be-havior than are police officers and social workers" (p. 21). Ennis and Siegel base their conclusions in part on the facts and failure of psychiatrists' predictions of dangerousness in Operation Bax-strom. Again, a quote from their book:

A famous example is the so-called Operation Baxstrom. In New York in 1966 there were almost 1,000 mentally ill exconvicts whom psychiatrists had examined and certified as being so danger-ous that they could not be accommodated in regular civil mental hospitals. The psychiatrists predicted that they could only be han-dled in high-security mental hospitals run by the Department of

Correction. Nevertheless, because of a Supreme Court decision (*Baxstrom* v. *Herold*), all of those patients were transferred to civil mental hospitals. Because the psychiatrists had predicted that those patients would be unusually dangerous, the employees of the civil hospitals threatened to resign and demanded higher wages. The psychiatric predictions turned out to be almost 100 percent wrong. After one year the Department of Mental Hygiene reported that "there have been no significant problems with the patients. All have been absorbed into the general patient population, many reside on open wards, over 200 have been released, and only seven have been certified as too dangerous for a civil hospital.

So, out of almost 1,000 predictions, the psychiatrists were right only seven times. They would have done better flipping coins. (pp. 21–22)

Although Operation Baxstrom may be an extreme case of the inaccuracy of psychiatric predictions of dangerousness, a summary of studies on predictions of violence (Rappaport, 1977) indicates that the behavioral sciences are very far from giving accurate predictions in general, and especially in specific instances. In fact, the behavioral sciences are at primitive levels when it comes to identifying accurately a truly dangerous person. Yet two assumptions, *erroneous* assumptions as the facts bear out, continue to linger: they are (a) that the mentally ill, as a group, are potentially dangerous, and (b) that mental health professionals can make accurate predictions of dangerousness and hence can be called as "expert witnesses" in giving testimony as to dangerousness.

Regarding the first point, the assumption that the mentally ill are a potentially dangerous group, Livermore, Malmquist, and Meehl (1968) have noted that other groups—for example, repeated speeding violators and drunk drivers—are potentially far more dangerous than most mental patients. As Ennis and Siegel point out, "We know that 85 percent of all convicted criminals will commit additional crimes after they are discharged from prison. But when their sentences expire, we let them go" (p. 23). Ennis and Litwack (1974) write that "there is no support in the literature for the popularly held notion that the mentally ill are more dangerous, as a group, than the general population, or for any belief that the presence of a psychiatric disturbance, per se, makes the prediction of violence easier and more accurate than would otherwise be the case" (p. 716). Yet the belief exists in most communities and courts that the mentally ill person is a danger, and this had led to the *presumption* of danger in many court cases (Kittrie, 1971; Scheff, 1973). After studying the commitment procedures in a midwestern state, Scheff (1973) came to the conclusion that the presumption of dangerousness is part of the general presumption of illness, which leads, in most cases, to courts and communities "playing it safe" — that is, hospitalizing — rather than running the risk that a released patient will do violence to himself or others. Scheff cites political reasons, as well as financial and ideological, for maintaining the presumptions of illness and dangerousness: judges are often elected officials and take their cue from community sentiment; and most communities (a) blanch at the headlines (or thought) of exmental patients doing violence, (b) blame the judiciary for the occurrence or fear of violence occurring, and (c) back up their feelings at the voting booth. Judges, recognizing that community rather than patient sentiment swings more votes,[6] often yield to the sentiments of the larger voting constituency — even if the belief that the sentiment is founded upon is erroneous.

It must be added that mental health professionals *share* the bias with the courts and communities regarding the potential dangerousness of mental patients. Monahan (1976) has reviewed the literature on prevention of violence and he finds in five studies in addition to Operation Baxstrom that professionals consistently and *vastly* overpredict violence.

There is also the second *erroneous* assumption, that behavioral scientists in general, and the mental health professionals in particular, can make accurate predictions. How did the assumption come to be? It might be well here to recite Robinson's (1973) remarks about "currying a bad press": Robinson makes the point that the press has been all too favorable to the behavioral sciences, and he perceives the danger that "the public will think we know what we are doing instead of appreciating the experimental nature of our enterprise" (p. 133). We are getting caught in court on our overblown press releases; in fact, we cannot deliver on our promises to predict dangerousness accurately. Kozol, Boucher, and Garofalo (1972) tell us that "No tests or psychiatric examinations can dependably predict a probability of dangerous behavior in the absence of an actual history of a severely violent assault on another person." The psychiatrist will look to past acts if there is no current evidence of violence, thus following the clinical maxim that *the best predictor of future acts is past acts.*

Even with a past violent act, however, our predictions are very far from "sure things." Many cases exist in which a violent act is committed without a prior, violent act. What then?

---

[6] Ennis and Siegel (1973) noted that a few years ago at least 36 states had laws that restrict the voting rights of mental patients.

How have we done at prediction? As Rappaport (1977) states:

The very procedures that allow for the involvement of mental health professionals in the system as predictors of dangerousness were introduced as a means to make the system more, rather than less, just for the individual offender. *What may need to be recognized is that the experiment is a failure.* Individual prediction is simply not accurate enough to be permitted, and it is the responsibility of mental health professionals and other social scientists to keep the public informed of this fact (p. 339).

Both Robinson (1973) and Rappaport (1977) are psychologists, judging the "competency of their science"; they are also noting societal, press, and judicial misjudgments of our competency. The danger exists that the wrong persons, the mental health professional and allegedly mentally ill patient, will be judged competent and incompetent, respectively.

Livermore and his associates (1968) explain part of the problem in statistical terms. Here is an example (Rappaport, 1977, p. 336) taken from their paper:

Livermore et al., have argued that because dangerous behavior is of very low incidence in society (e.g., the number of people who will actually kill, rape, and so on, is small relative to the number who will not), any test of dangerousness must be applied to a large number of people. To isolate those who are dangerous it is necessary to incarcerate many who are not. They provide the following example: Assume that 1 of 1000 persons is dangerous to self or others and that a test identifying these persons is 95 percent accurate (there are no psychological tests or other methods shown to be anything near this accurate). If 100,000 people were screened, 95 out of 100 who are dangerous would be identified, five would be missed, but of the 99,900 who are not dangerous, 4995 would be called dangerous when they are not.

If, in the criminal law, it is better that ten guilty men go free than that one innocent man suffer, how can we say in the civil commitment area that it is better that fifty-four harmless people be incarcerated lest one dangerous man be free? (Livermore, Malmquist, & Meehl, 1968, p. 84)

Scott and Ennis, in an *Amicus Curiae* brief (1975, p. 8) submitted on behalf of the American Orthopsychiatric Association in *Mathew* v. *Nelson,* quote from an American Psychiatric Association published *Task Force Report 8: Clinical Aspects of the Violent Individual.* The report states that "neither psychiatrists nor anyone else have reliably demonstrated an ability to predict future violence of 'dangerousness.' Neither has any special psychiatric 'expertise' in this area been established." Ennis and Litwack (62

Calif. L. Rev. 693, 1974), in a paper entitled "Psychiatry and the Presumption of Expertise: Flipping Coins in the Courtroom," point out that "Unlike the task of formulating a diagnosis, psychiatrists are not even trained in the assessment or prediction of dangerousness. Medical schools do not offer courses in the prediction of dangerous behavior; nor are there textbooks explaining the method and criteria by which such assessments are to be made" (p. 733). If this is the true state of the science (of psychiatry, prediction, and the medical school curriculum), and Ennis and Litwack assert it is, then why should psychiatrists be permitted to testify as experts in civil commitment proceedings? The authors conclude that they do not qualify as expert witnesses. They conclude their paper by citing the 1964 words of a judge, now Chief Justice Warren E. Burger,[7] who wrote (pp. 751-752) that "psychology is, at best, an 'infant among the family of science,' that psychiatry and psychology cannot claim to be truly scientific, and that psychiatrists and psychologists may be claiming too much in relation to what they really understand about the human personality and human behavior." The professional literature confirms Justice Berger's intuitive judgment; psychiatrists have bitten off more than they can chew. The fault, however, is not theirs alone, for legislatures and courts, in an attempt to shift responsibility for making the determination of who shall remain free and who shall be confined, have turned to psychiatry, seeking easy answers where there are none.

Human behavior is difficult to understand, and, at present, impossible to predict at the level of certainty claimed by physicists for balls rolling down inclined planes. People do not behave that unidirectionally. So, subject to constitutional limitations, the decision to deprive another human of liberty is not so much a psychiatric judgment as it is a social judgment. We shall have to decide how much we value individual freedom; how much we care about privacy and self-determination; how much deviance we can tolerate — or how much suffering. There are no "experts" to make those decisions for us.

INTO THE "VOID FOR VAGUENESS"

"Dangerous?" What does it mean? Dangerous to whom? To what?

If a husband threatens to throw his wife's precious china heirloom into the air, or if she threatens to use his stamp collection to mail out chain letters, can the threatened destruction of

---

[7] Burger, Psychiatrists, Lawyers, and the Courts, 28 Fed. Prob. 3, 7, (1964).

property be cited as fitting the "dangerous" criterion, and thus serve as grounds for involuntary hospitalization? Ennis and Siegel (1973) state, "In some states (Montana and New Jersey, for example) a person can be hospitalized if, in the absence of hospitalization, he would (or might) cause damage to property" (p. 20). Does threatened property damage seem like a sensible criterion to justify the loss of liberty? Does this judgment depend, ultimately, on the *value* of the property, with the appraiser holding the final word on commitment?

How serious, and imminent, is the threat? We have already seen that laymen and professionals tend to overestimate the seriousness and imminence of potentially dangerous situations. Would they likewise overestimate the potential danger to property? These and related questions are only beginning to be addressed by the courts. A case in the United State District Court for the District of Hawaii, *Suzuki* v. *Yuen* (1977), addressed the danger to property criterion (46 LW 2181). The judge found that nonvoluntary commitment on grounds of dangerous to property violates the due process clause of the Fourteenth Amendment. The judge wrote:

> Recent authorities require a specific finding of dangerousness to self or others before commitment may occur, and thus impliedly exclude dangerousness to property as a basis for hospitalization. I believe the requirements of substantive due process are met only when an individual is found to be dangerous to himself or to others, and thus hold that dangerousness to property is not a constitutional basis for commitment in an emergency or nonemergency situation.
>
> The state's interest is not so compelling to justify commitment on any other basis, especially where the state's interest can be adequately protected through the use of criminal statutes prohibiting damage to property.

If the Hawaii decision is the new bellwether, then judicial winds are blowing toward alleged patient rights, safeguards, and protections; whether the weather continues to be this favorable for the allegedly mentally ill patient, or turns unseasonable, remains to be seen. A trend is becoming discernible though: the divestment process — excluding certain groups and actions from criminal proceedings and safeguards in favor of civil proceedings and less protections — may have peaked, and what we are witnessing now are the ebb tides.

Regarding dangerousness, we can move from property to persons, yet the ambiguity over what is dangerous lingers. What does "dangerous to himself or others" mean? Ennis and Siegel

(1973) highlight the definitional ambiguity in the following quote: "Some psychiatrists consider a person 'dangerous to himself' if he does not eat balanced meals or if he smokes too much, and 'dangerous to others' if he talks too loudly in public places or if he bombards public officials with letters complaining about real or imagined grievances" (p. 20).

Two points emerge. First, the term "dangerous" is dangerously frought with ambiguity. The statutes in many states are sufficiently imprecise as written that lawyers have challenged the standard on "void-for-vagueness" grounds. "Voids," they argue, allow too much free play for fears, biases, projections, mischievousness, and malevolence to be acted out. Ennis and Siegel (1973) comment on the legal challenge, and voice their recommendations:

> Whether that challenge would succeed would depend on the exact wording of the statute being challenged, and on the attitudes and philosophy of the judges who decide the case. Some judges believe that hospitalization statutes must be just as precise as "criminal" statutes, but others disagree. There are very few court decisions on this issue and it is impossible to predict what the courts will do in the future. But no lawyer, and no patient, should be satisfied with the wording of the "danger" standard in his state unless it is at least as precise as the standards in California and Massachusetts.
>
> In California, a person is considered dangerous to himself only if he "threatened or attempted to take his own life," and dangerous to others only if he presents an "imminent threat of substantial physical harm to others." The statute thus specifies the *type* of danger (physical harm), the *degree* of danger (substantial), and the *time period* within which the danger is thought likely to occur (imminent).
>
> In Massachusetts, a person is considered dangerous only if he (1) has threatened or attempted suicide or (2) has exhibited actual homicidal or violent behavior. (pp. 22–23)

The second point to emerge is that the danger standard, when applied, is a form of *preventive detention*; it deprives one of liberty on the basis of a *potential, future act,* and not on what someone did. Preventive detention is punishment without a crime; looked at this way, the concept and its employment rankles our democratic sense of fairness; and looked at another way, it itself is a crime — the crime of punishment without crime. In fact, in the most celebrated, preventive detention case in recent years, the massive arrest of May Day demonstrators, the courts awarded monetary damages for the wrongful prevention detention of over 1000 demonstrators. Yet, we consider and still countenance preventive detention when it comes to psychiatric patients who are alleged to be potentially dangerous. What is the difference? What accounts for the *un*equal protection under law of this group?

The question turns on "mental illness." Let me use Ennis and Siegel (1973) again to set forth the issue:

> The point is simple. If a person is sane, he cannot be deprived of liberty because of what he might do in the future, no matter how dangerous we may think he is. We know that 85 percent of all convicted criminals will commit additional crimes after they are discharged from prison. But when their sentences expire, we let them go. On the other hand, if a person (including an exprisoner) is thought to be insane, he can then be deprived of liberty because of what he might do in the future. Why should that be? Why should we prohibit preventive detention of the sane but permit preventive detention of the insane? (p. 23)

In Thomas Szasz's essay (1970), "Involuntary Mental Hospitalization: A Crime Against Humanity," he mentions alternatives to involuntary hospitalization and its preventive detention aspect:

> Although psychiatric methods of coercion are indisputably useful for those who employ them, they are clearly not indispensable for dealing with the problems that so-called mental patients pose for those about them. If an individual threatens others by virtue of his beliefs or actions, he could be dealt with by methods other than "medical": if his conduct is ethically offensive, moral sanctions against him might be appropriate; if forbidden by law, legal sanctions might be appropriate. In my opinion, both informal, moral sanctions, such as social ostracism or divorce, and formal, judicial sanctions, such as fine and imprisonment, are more dignified and less injurious to the human spirit than the quasi-medical psychiatric sanction of involuntary mental hospitalization. (p. 119)

For now it is enough to raise the questions and suggest that there may be alternatives. In the next section on nonemergency hospitalization, the issue of preventive detention will be discussed more thoroughly.

NONEMERGENCY HOSPITALIZATION

Emergency commitment procedures are designed to *protect* citizens from suspected mentally ill people who might be potentially dangerous; the commitment is usually for a brief period of time (e.g., 48 hours, 5 days, 15 days) and ostensibly for *observation and diagnosis*. Nonemergency hospitalization procedures are invoked to *help* the prospective patient; as such, their focus is *treatment*. As examples of nonemergency standards, Oregon requires that examiners find the person "mentally ill and in need of treatment, care, or custody," Ohio uses "mentally ill and in need of care and treatment," and Oklahoma mentions, in part, "mental illness and the incapability of managing himself or his affairs." The length of stay for nonemergency hospitalization is considerably longer than emergency procedures (e.g., 90 days in Ohio), with indefinite hospitalization sanctioned in many states (Ennis & Siegel, 1973). Because of the indefinite or long-term loss of freedom that results from this paternalistic hospitalization (i.e., Mill's harm principle is not invoked but the prospective patient's best interests are), it is important to scrutinize the steps, rationales, and results involved — but first, its history.

We have already seen (Foucault, 1973) commitment sanctioned for reasons other than imminent dangerousness in the classical age of the seventeenth and eighteenth centuries. The poor, the mendicants, prodigal sons, the debauched or soon-to-be debauched, blasphemers, the unbaptized, who refused a watery immersion and a spiritual birth, and those who aired themselves by strolling the cities in their birthday suits, all were likely candidates for *lettres de cachet* and commitment.

The first judicial endorsement of this "broadened" commitment criteria in "the name of therapy" was alleged to have been made by Chief Justice Shaw of Massachusetts in 1845,[8] where he "ruled that restraint of the insane was legally justified not only by regard for public or personal safety, but by consideration of remedial treatment. This was probably the first time that the therapeutic justification for restraint was explicitly stated in a decision handed down by an American court" (Deutsch, 1949, p. 423). However, Kittrie (1971) points out in a footnote to Deutsch's quote that "the cited case contains no clear expression of such a proposition. The paucity of legal critiques in the *parens patriae* area is well illustrated by the continued reliance upon this lone and ambiguous case as a landmark decision in the growth of therapeutic commitment powers" (p. 66). Whether it was explicit or only implied by Chief Justice Shaw, it is clear from a reading of legal history following 1845 that states did broaden their commitment statutes such that "need for treatment" became sufficient grounds for commitment. In fact, as Kittrie (1971) points

---

[8] In *re* Josiah Oakes, 8 Law Rep. 122 (Mass. 1845).

out, "Some states have even made the welfare needs of persons other than the patient, such as members of his family, a sufficient criterion for commitment" (p. 67).

As the law broadens, so, it seems, does its reach. Kittrie cites figures for 1949 that reveal that almost 90% of admissions to state mental hospitals were involuntary.[9] Ennis and Siegel (1973) give figures for 1963 of 80% of admissions being involuntary, and although the figures have lowered considerably since then—that is, there being a growing consciousness concerning involuntary commitments and their abuse and failures, along with a greater effort to reduce their use in favor of voluntary admissions—much of this recent lowering results from newer ligation and rulings. The winds of judicial rulings seem to be swinging toward patient "rights," such as the "right to treatment" cases of recent years (*Donaldson*[10] and *Wyatt*[11] cases). But winds are shifty and intangible, as shifty as a point of view and as tangible as a moment of consciousness; yet it is the consciousness underlying these historical and judicial happenings that bears scrutiny—along with the dramas of the men who enact them. We now move to the drama of a nonemergency hospitalization commitment hearing.

NOTICE

Because nonemergency involuntary commitment procedures are considered *civil* rather than *criminal,* full "due process" guarantees that are granted citizens in criminal proceedings may be diminished in a civil hearing. "Notice" is one such diminished guarantee. Some states require that notice be given to the patient prior to judicial action, whereas other states deny notice, or ignore the question; and the United States Supreme Court has not ruled on whether "an alleged mentally ill person is constitutionally entitled to prior notice" (Kittrie, 1971, p. 84).

Ennis and Siegel (1973) argue for notice:

> The prospective patient should be given written notice of the purpose, time, and place of the hearing, and he should be notified sufficiently in advance of the hearing to enable him to prepare for it. The notice should specify the statutory basis for the proceeding and should tell the prospective patient exactly what he has done or said that suggests he is mentally ill or dangerous. (p. 33)

This, I assume, includes emergency and nonemergency involuntary commitments.

[9] *O'Connor* v. *Donaldson,* 422 U.S. 563 (1975).

[11] *Wyatt* v. *Stickney,* 325 F. Supp. 781, 784 (M.D. Ala. 1971).

A number of psychiatrists have argued against notice (Kittrie, 1971) for disturbed individuals. One point that has been raised is the potential traumatic effect (i.e., producing anxiety and confusion) notice can have. Besides the danger of psychological trauma, some feel that notice would not produce the hoped for "understanding," since the person is not mentally capable of understanding the nature of the proceedings.

Kittrie (1971) rebuts the "lack of understanding" argument against notice in the following quote: "To decide that a person is too deranged to benefit from notice, moreover, is effectively to prejudge his competency. Said the Kansas Court of Appeals:[12] 'It will not do to say it is useless to serve notice upon an insane person; that it would avail nothing because of his inability to take advantage of it. His sanity is the very thing to be tried' " (p. 85).

Returning to the first point, that of potential psychic trauma, it will not do to say that the effect of notice is always psychologically traumatic. What could be more traumatic than suddenly finding yourself in a mental hospital without warning? Can a person's sense of betrayal, powerlessness, and rage be assuaged by telling him, belatedly, "that we did it in your best interests—so you would not be traumatized"?

"Would we accept these words for ourselves if the shoes were suddenly reversed?" My suspicion would be that I would cry: "Why aren't you being honest with me?" "What happened to Mill's 'persuading and remonstrating'?" and other words, more affective, less intellectualized.

On the other side, to re-reverse shoes for the moment, I would be hard pressed to justify my *deception*: Why was I avoiding the confrontation with him, myself, my beliefs, and my illusions? To tell myself that notice would only arouse him, cause more agitation in him and the family, lead more likely to dangerous behavior (*my* prediction, please recognize, and likely to be overrated if I am like most professionals)—and thus, should be avoided—just will not do, ethically and therapeutically. I cannot send someone to a hospital to get help—for example, therapy—a process that in its best and classical sense is one of self-discovery ("to know thyself") conducted with a pledge of self-honesty [see Freud's (1953) 1913 paper, "Further Recommendations in the Technique of Psychoanalysis"], if I am not being honest *in the process*. "How can this process begin on a note of dishonesty?" "If I do not 'level' about my intentions, will he?" "If I enact the very behavior and consciousness I want him to change, will he?"

---

[12] In *re* Willman, 3 Kan. App. 100, 103, 45 P. 726, 727 (1896).

No, this will not do. It is not even good therapy. If you believe in a particular case that commitment would be in the person's best therapeutic interest, it means, to me, that you ultimately want him to confront his own behavior and beliefs, be they delusional thoughts or bizzare acts. Notice seems to put him on notice that that public accounting will occur. If the alleged patient has another point of view, it affords him the time to present that point for all "to see." "Can a complete look hurt more than a purposefully incomplete one?" This therapist does not believe it does, in therapy or in court. "Can one or the other be treated with less honesty and justice?"

That a commitment hearing is likely to be unpleasant goes without saying; it can well be traumatic for *all* concerned: prospective patients, family members, mental health professionals, lawyers, and judges. All may experience "anxiety and confusion" and be shook to their roots in this drama. A drama this potent is a "character test" for all. Our fears, hurts, and anguish, along with countermeasures to deny, project, isolate, and intellectualize may all come out in our actions and words. So will our ethics, in our conduct of this drama.

COUNSEL

Is the perspective patient entitled to be represented by a lawyer, and should the court appoint a free lawyer if he can not afford one? Ennis and Siegel (1973) ask the following question, "Is the appointment of a lawyer automatic?" and answer as follows:

> Generally, no. Even if the patient or prospective patient has a *right* to a free lawyer, most states will not give him one unless he affirmatively demands that a lawyer be assigned. That is a strange rule of law. It places upon a person alleged to be mentally incapable of caring for himself the affirmative burden of protecting his interests by demanding the appointment of a lawyer. Persons charged with crime do not have to demand lawyers. If they are poor, they are automatically assigned lawyers, whether they ask for them or not. Furthermore, alleged criminals are not permitted to "waive" or give up their right to a lawyer unless the court finds that the waiver was "knowingly and intelligently" made.
>
> For prospective patients the rule is just the opposite. Unless they affirmatively demand a lawyer they will be presumed to have waived their right to counsel.

Kittrie (1971) (p. 41) makes the following comments:

> What should be the function of counsel in a mental commitment proceeding? A 1961 American Bar Foundation report notes that

counsel must guard not only against scheming relatives but also against incompetent and lax medical judgment and the improper extension of involuntary commitments to borderline cases. He must make certain that a patient's need for treatment not be denied merely because of his inability to pay for hospitalization. Counsel's role extends not only to the protection of the patient's liberty, but also to the safeguarding of his property. The court may need to be alerted to the advisability of declaring a patient incompetent and appointing a guardian to protect real and personal property. Counsel can help the patient meet the legal–economic problems that might arise as a consequence of institutionalization, such as family support, overdue installment payments, and possible property foreclosures. Counsel can effectively contribute to a reduction in the use of involuntary commitments by making certain that other community alternatives are fully explored and utilized and by persuading patients who require hospital care to choose voluntary institutionalization over compulsory treatment.

Perhaps the main task of legal counsel, in this as in the other realms of the therapeutic state, is the "individualizing function" — insistence upon careful, fair, and personalized assessment of every case in the face of depersonalized people-processing bureaucracies. One recent commentator thus portrays the attorney as the possible possessor of the key for unlocking the "closed circuitry of decision making" in the modern therapeutic state. (pp. 92–93)

Counsel can have quite an effect. The study by Wenger and Fletcher (1973) on "The Effect of Legal Counsel on Admissions to a State Mental Hospital: A Confrontation of Professions" amply confirms this. They studied 81 cases, 15 represented by counsel and 66 having no legal counsel. The average length of time for the hearing was 8.13 minutes. If you had counsel, however, the hearing was likely to be longer; in fact, the hearings averaged more than twice as long as those in which legal counsel was not present. But more important than time is the admission decision. Without legal counsel, 91% of the cases were admitted; with legal counsel, only 26% were admitted. Now it is possible that this huge and significant difference is, in part or whole, spurious: perhaps the "sane" person is more likely to acquire legal counsel than the "insane" person, thus the two groups might not be matched to begin with. To control for this possibility, Wenger and Fletcher had independent observers rate the prepatients on judgment, self-control, need for guidance, dangerousness, and the like. They then grouped these ratings, using three categories: commitment criteria met, borderline, and commitment criteria not met. Their analysis revealed that "legal counsel affects the admission of patients within each condition. . . . From the above data it appears that the inverse relationship between the presence of legal counsel and mental hospital admissions is not spurious. Lawyers do appear to lessen the likelihood of their clients being admitted" (p. 143).

The legal profession and the medical profession confront each other at commitment hearings. They come to it from different points of view that can clash sharply.

First, the medical profession favors "easy" commitment procedures. The profession believes that the needs of the patient are best met by allowing for rapid placement in the mental hospital without legal qualifications. For example, the doctors believe that (1) rules of evidence exclude much that is medically relevant, (2) the atmosphere of the courtroom has a punitive aura, (3) the terminology of the law is traumatic to sensitive people, (4) excessive legalism discourages families from seeking early medical care, etc. The legal profession, on the other hand, favors "strict" commitment. Lawyers believe that the individual's civil liberties are best served if the due process of the law is *not* removed. (Wenger & Fletcher, 1973, pp. 136–7)

Although I disagree with the overgeneralization – that the medical profession favors "easy" commitment whereas the legal profession favors "strict" (to me, it is not that clear and distinct) – I do favor the *dialogue*. The dialogue, which once did flourish, fell into silence once the reason–madness nexus became rooted in our consciousness (Foucault, 1973):

In the serene world of mental illness, modern man no longer communicates with the madman: on one hand, the man of reason delegates the physican to madness, thereby authorizing a relation only through the abstract universality of disease; . . . As for a common language, there is no such thing; or rather, there is no such thing any longer; the constitution of madness as a mental illness, at the end of the eighteenth century, affords the evidence of a broken dialogue, posits the separation as already effected, and thrusts into oblivion all those stammered, imperfect words without fixed syntax in which the exchange between madness and reason was made. The language of psychiatry, which is a monologue of reason *about* madness, has been established only on the basis of such a silence. (pp. x–x11)

The silence needs to be broken; the dialogue must resume; and the courtroom, not just the therapist's office or hospital ward, is the place for the airing, the public airing, of disagreements. This is the direction that the Task Panel of the President's Commission on Mental Health (1978) recommends: they present the case for an advocacy perspective, and recommend the establishment of an adequately financed system of comprehensive advocacy services for mentally handicapped persons. Protection and advocacy are needed from someone "outside" the circle of family, friends, and doctors who has the facility for entering the courtroom and dialoguing. The courtroom encounter reestablishes a dialogue between medical psychology and law, and between prospective patient and family. The dialogue, as Plato penned and Socrates enacted (those Hellenic revealers of law, ethics, and psychology), was the way of education, enlightenment, and right conduct. After all, is not that precisely what we are seeking now?

THE OPPORTUNITY TO BE HEARD AND TO CROSS-EXAMINE

I am advocating, like others before me (Ennis & Siegel, 1973; Kittrie, 1971), that the alleged patient be given an opportunity to be heard. Not only to be heard, but to cross-examine doctors, family members, or others who submit evidence that might form the basis for the hospitalization decision. This is no more than a criminal proceeding guarantees. Because the loss of liberty can be as great as in criminal cases, if not greater (*indefinite* hospitalization), the procedural steps and due process guarantees ought to be equivalent. Being heard is not always easy, especially when the closing judicial gavel falls before the echo from the opening gavel clears. (Scheff (1973), who examined the judicial hearing in a midwestern state, found that the hearings were conducted with "lightning rapidity," with the mean time of the hearings being 1.6 minutes. The alleged patient should be allowed to clear his throat before he is cleared from the courtroom. He should be allowed to call witnesses in his own behalf. As to whether he is entitled, if he is indigent, to free expert witnesses, remains to be litigated. My point and question (to be answered more fully in a subsequent section) is more psychological and factual than legal: Does the psychiatrist or psychologist deserve the adjective "expert"? If it turns out that "there are no experts," then the legal question of a right to free expert witnesses becomes moot.

PROTECTION AGAINST SELF-INCRIMINATION

The Fifth Amendment grants us the privilege against self-incrimination; we can remain silent in exercising that right and suffer no penalty. But what if mental illness is alleged? If, during a prehearing psychiatric examination, one chooses to remain silent, can he be penalized?

Before answering this, let us examine the silence from a psychiatrist's point of view. The psychiatrist has been sent to a hospital by the court to determine the alleged patient's "mental status." Although a mental status examination may cover (a) appearance and behavior, (b) speech, (c) mood, (d) thought content, (e) perception, (f) orientation as to time, space, and person, (g) attention and concentration, (h) memory (both recent and past), (i) information, (j) vocabulary, (k) abstraction, and (1) judgment and comprehension, when it is performed for the courts it is usually more abbreviated; in fact, Scheff (1973) reports that in his study of court-employed psychiatirc examinations, the mean time for the interview was 9.2 minutes. Scheff noted that two lines of questioning seemed routine: the first concerned the circumstances that led to the patient's hospitalization, and the second focused on the patient's orientation and capacity for abstract thinking.

Now, if that patient refuses to answer, what might the psychiatrist think regarding this lack of cooperativeness? Perhaps the patient's refusal is a way of hiding a sensorial defect. Perhaps it is a manifestation of a guarded, suspicious personality. Might it be seen as defensive, or paranoid? What I am saying is that the silence may be seen as a *symptom* rather than a *right*. It may be "confirmatory evidence" for mental illness.

Recently the United States District Court for the District of Hawaii[13] examined a statute (H. R. S. SS 334-(b)(4)(G) which permitted the hospitalization of a person in a nonemergency situation in which the individual refused participation in a precommitment psychiatric examination. Here we have the case of someone temporarily committed against his will, as the district judge wrote, "precisely because he chooses to exercise his constitutional right to remain silent." The decision goes on to read:

The Fifth and Fourteenth amendments secure "the right of a person to remain silent unless he chooses to speak in the unfettered exercise of his own will, and to suffer no penalty . . . for such silence." . . . The Supreme Court has held that individuals may not be coerced into waiving their right to remain silent by being penalized for asserting it. . . .

SS 334-(b)(4)(G) penalizes an individual who chooses to exercise his Fifth Amendment right by temporarily hospitalizing him contrary to his will. Because the statute has the effect of coercing an individual to waive a constitutional right, it is unconstitutional under the Fourteenth Amendment.

It is recommended that this right against self-incrimination

---

[13] *Suzuki* v. *Yuen*, (Civil No. 73-3854, 1977).

be extended to prospective patients; after all, it is only giving *them* what *we* already possess. And is not that beneficence at its best? Let the irony not be lost: we would not be giving them anything if we had not taken it away — taken it away under the presumption that there is a "we" and a "them." Maybe I am recommending far more than a legal extension of a basic right. I am recommending that we seek to close the reason–madness nexus between "we" and "them," and within a consciousness that produces "we and them" thinking. I would like to thank Erasmus for that timely suggestion.

PROOF BEYOND A REASONABLE DOUBT

In nonemergency hospitalization hearings, judgments as to mental illness or health and need for treatment or not are rendered. How much doubt in our judgment can we live with if the consequence for the alleged patient is his loss of freedom? What degree of confidence should we require in our judgments? Some states require proof "beyond a reasonable doubt," which is the standard in criminal proceedings (Ennis & Siegel, 1973). However, many states require less proof: it may be a "preponderance of evidence," or "sufficient evidence," or a "majority of the evidence." Some recent court cases (*Suzuki* v. *Quisenberry*[14], Proctor v. *Butler*[15], *In Re Ballay*[16]) have addressed this issue. Appel (1973) presents a legal analysis of *In Re Ballay*:

> What standard of proof should be required to deprive an individual of his freedom? Should the answer depend upon the specific grounds on which society seeks to confine a person? The United States Court of Appeals for the District of Columbia Circuit has just recently considered these due process issues within the context of involuntary civil commitment. In *In Re Ballay* the court concluded that regardless of the reason behind institutionalization, the magnitude of individual interests at stake requires the same standard of proof as that needed to imprison. (p. 409)

The argument in *In Re Ballay* was an extention of the Supreme Court finding in *In Re Winship*,[17] which "held that a juvenile, charged in a juvenile proceeding with an act that would constitute a crime if committed by an adult, must be afforded a standard of proof beyond a reasonable doubt as one of the essentials of due process. Underlying *Winship* is the concept that when individual liberty is at stake, procedural safeguards must duly

---

[14] *Suzuki* v. *Quisenberry,* 411 F. Supp. 1113, 44 LW2422 (1976).

[15] *Proctor* v. *Butler,* N.H. Sup. Ct., (1977).

[16] *In Re Ballay,* 482 F 2d 648 (D.C. Cir. 1973).

reflect and provide for this immense concern unless weightier interests work to qualify this general principle" (Appel, 1973, p. 411). Does the state's role as *parens patriae* qualify as a weightier qualifier of this general principle? Appel argues that it does not. He reminds the reader of Justice Brandeis' dissenting comments in *Olmstead* v. *United States*:[18] "Experience should teach us to be most on our guard to protect liberty when the Government's purposes are beneficent. Men born to freedom are naturally alert to repel invasion of their liberty by evil-minded rulers. The greatest dangers to liberty lurk in insidious encroachment by men of zeal, well-meaning but without understanding" (p. 412).

In the Hawaii case (*Suzuki* v. *Quisenberry*, Note 14), the plaintiff challenged the temporary commitment of an individual when the commitment was based on the "sufficient evidence" rather than on "proof beyond a reasonable doubt" standard, whereas the defendants argued that "sufficient evidence" was a proper standard since that confinement was of a temporary, rather than indefinite, duration. The judge ruled for the plaintiff, invoked *In Re Ballay,* and wrote that because "an individual's liberty is an interest of transcending value," one ought to demand a greater "quantum of proof" than "sufficient evidence" provides; thus proof beyond a reasonable doubt was accepted as the standard in that instance.

A similar ruling resulted in *Proctor* v. *Butler* (Note 15) such that the due process guarantees of New Hampshire constitution require the "beyond reasonable doubt" standard of proof to be used in involuntary commitment proceedings.

This seems to be the direction in which the legal winds are blowing these days; as a result, alleged patients are being granted greater protections, and civil proceedings are coming to mirror criminal proceedings more and more. I would applaud, had not the lessons of history tempered my exuberance. As history amply confirms, legal winds shift. The winds may reverse again. Yet whatever the current breezes and their legal justifications may be, my concern is chiefly with the underlying spirit and psychology that moves them. It is the psychological implications and entanglements, and how they may involve or ensnare the mental health professional, that is the central thread of this book. Let us follow and examine the psychological processes underlying the issues of certainty and doubt.

Certainty of proof is hinged to facts, but facts are often hard

---

[17] *In Re Winship,* 397 U.S. 358 (1970).
[18] *Olmstead* v. *United States,* 277 U.S. 438, a479 (1928).

to come by in questions of mental illness; and "facts," on closer examination, often turn out to be "expert opinions" (i.e., the opinions of psychiatrists and clinical psychologists based on interviews or tests), which are often at *odds* with one another. Citing from *The United States Law Week* (46 LW 2285, 12/6/77) in reference to *Proctor* v. *Butler* (Note 15), they write, "If anything, the predictive nature of the ultimate finding and the frequently conflicting opinions of psychiatric experts reinforce the court's determination to impose a standard of proof that will ensure the utmost care in reaching an involuntary commitment decision."

If it is true that psychiatric experts fail to agree and have "reasonable doubts" with one another in terms of diagnosing, predicting, and treating the alleged patient's behavior, then the alleged patient ought to be protected from our judgments to the utmost degree, or beyond reasonable doubt. Let us examine our "reasonable doubts"—their extent, roots, and reasons. This task is important since decisions regarding liberty hang on these judgments. In fact, Scheff (1973) tells us that psychiatric testimony at commitment hearings is given the greatest weight in decision making; although judges are given the final decision and responsibility regarding commitment, they rarely release an alleged patient if it was not recommended by the psychiatrist following psychiatric examination. Given the import of psychiatric judgments, it is important to examine the literature on the reliability and validity of psychiatric diagnoses.

RELIABILITY

"Reliability" usually refers to the frequency or probability of agreement between two or more independent observers when answering the same question. For example, the questions might be, "Is Mr. A mentally ill?" "What is Mr. A's diagnosis?" "Will involuntary hospitalization and treatment aid the patient?" Reliability figures can be computed for each question, but typically, in the reliability literature, only the first two questions are addressed (Ennis & Litwack, 1974). When these questions have been addressed in reliability studies, the results, in general, have been disappointing (Arthur, 1969; Buss, 1966; Zigler & Phillips, 1961). In one of the first and most widely cited studies, Ash (1949) measured the diagnostic agreement between two or three psychiatrists after they had jointly interviewed 52 patients. For specific diagnoses, there was agreement among the three psychiatrists in 21% of the cases, and total disagreement in 31% of the cases. The broad categories of disorder showed limited reliability, but the specific categories were hardly reliable at all. Schmidt and Fonda (1956) found more positive results: high reliability (92%) for organic brain syndromes, 80% agreement for nonorganic psychosis, and moderate reliability (71%) for nonpsychotic disturbances. When it came to specific diagnoses in the three broad categories, reliability fell to 55% agreement. Kreitman, Sainsbury, Morrissey, Towers, and Scrivener (1961) found the same trend: respectable agreement (78%) for generic categories, lesser agreement (63%) for specific diagnoses. In sum, the major, generic categories produced agreement that ranged from 58% to 84%, (organic syndromes showing higher reliability than psychoses, which were higher than neuroses), whereas specific categories showed reliability that ranged from 34% to 63%. It ought to be noted that controlled (laboratory) studies, of which the above cited studies are examples, usually yield higher reliability than diagnostic practices "in the field." In laboratory studies, psychiatrists often hear the same interview, and they may talk with each other ahead of time to discuss various diagnostic categories, semantic confusions, and reach a consensus as to specific criteria (Ward, Beck, Mendelson, Mock, & Erbaugh, 1962); these attempts to improve reliability ratings are seldom present in everyday practices in the field.

Disappointing reliability figures have led many to abandon the current diagnostic schema and propose newer systems: some of the newer trends have favored a behavioral rather than a disease focus (Kanfer & Saslow, 1969), an emphasis on statistical rather than clinical, intuitive approaches (Meehl, 1956), computer and check-list symptom inventories rather than syndromes and methods of inference (Philips, Breverman, & Zigler, 1966; Smith, 1966), and decision-making models directed to consequences rather than directed to etiology (Arthur, 1969). The problems with reliability, the debate within the discipline, and the rash of "new, improved" models on the market to improve reliability are *symptomatic*. Judges, who are not clinicians by training and who may not be interested in the nuances of diagnostic labels, nomenclatures, and chi-squares tests, can recognize the *symptoms of disturbance* within a discipline. The symptoms are evident. Professionals within the discipline are questioning their own practices and proposing changes. Change rather than stability is the continued prognosis. We have not sorted out our own symptoms and systems. And when we have tried to sort "others," we have not agreed with each other on the sort, the reason for the sort, and the value of the sort. Let the courts beware! Over the last 100 years, the court and the mental health profession have courted one another, for different reasons, each looking to the other for answers and respectability that were not coming from within. Before the wedding is consummated, and before the inevitable "morning after" occurs, we ought to face honestly whether the promise made can be kept. For judgments based on unreliable practices may promise certainty, only to give way to doubt and illusion the morning after. My prenuptual advice is twofold, sincere, but somewhat trite: for the groom, the paternalistic professional, "demonstrate reliability before making vows"; for the blindfolded bride, the court, "look out."

VALIDITY

"Validity" refers to the accuracy of judgments: do they correlate with some facts in the external world? We have already examined one question, "Can psychiatrists accurately predict dangerousness?" and found psychiatric predictions to be invalid. Now let us examine the validity of predictions of mental illness. To set the question properly and appreciate its difficulties, an analogy is first drawn. Let us imagine that a man falls on his wrist and feels sharp, intense pain which persists for several days. His wrist swells up and turns blue. Two days later he thinks it may be a broken wrist. Is his diagnosis valid? To answer the question, we would want some type of confirmation or correlative finding in reality. An x-ray might be taken to reveal the presence of an underlying break. Although x-ray's are not perfect—that is they may miss detecting some breaks that are there or indicate a break when there is not one—the technology "seems accurate enough" for us, and medical science, to place faith in it. We may ask the analogous question regarding mental illness: does it correlate with some facts in the external world? For physical illnesses (e.g., the broken wrist), the symptoms have correlates within the physiological or anatomical (organic) reality; however, for mental illnesses, organic correlates to the overt symptoms are rarely found (Finkel, 1976) or mentioned;[19] this has led Szasz (1961), perhaps the most forceful critic of the "medical model," to label "mental illness" a *myth*. If there is no organic condition, there is no "illness."

If etiology of any kind (be it organic or psychological) is not specified, then we have a purely descriptive system of categorization. One possible problem with descriptive systems is to *assume*

[19] See Committee on Nomenclature and Statistics of the American Psychiatric Association, 1972, DSM-I or DSM-II. Most of the major categories of disorder specify no organic condition.

or attribute correlations when none in fact exist. We have already seen one assumed correlation that turned out to be erroneous — that the mentally ill are dangerous. If someone had the diagnosis "schizophrenia," some might assume that the schizophrenic was dangerous, incorrigible, unable to hold a job, and biologically defective; all of these stereotypes or assumed attributes, however widespread they may be, are not supported empirically.

Another problem with descriptive systems is when we assume that the label has *explanatory* power. A descriptive label does not. Saying someone is weird because they are schizophrenic says nothing. To say that his ambivalence, autism, affect, and associative disturbances are the result of schizophrenia is tautological: ambivalence, autism, affect, and associative disturbances are the defining characteristics of schizophrenia; thus making the substitution, we wind up saying, "He is schizophrenic because he is schizophrenic"; someone not versed in psychiatric terminology and "psychologic" might find that schizophrenic.

Validity and reliability in regard to the current *Diagnostic and Statistical Manual II* (Note 19) are further muddied by unclear phrases, similar symptoms for several disorders, definitional overlap between broad categories (Finkel, 1976), and "excessively fine distinctions" within broad categories (Ennis & Litwack, 1974). In addition to problems with the manual, there are problems with the professional and his practices. For example, the orientation and training of mental health professionals may create a set "to see" mental illness. Along with this, psychiatrists are often asked to judge illness or health within a context — the psychiatric hospital — that again favors the perception of illness: talking to a man in hospital pajamas, robe, and slippers, against the backdrop of a ward of patients, may bias the clinical judgment toward illness. Furthermore, the brevity of most psychiatric interviews (9.2 minutes according to Scheff, 1973), the fact that interviews are rarely repeated at future times (unless a judge specifically orders it), and the feelings of strangeness engendered by conversation where one's mental status is on the line may result in an insufficient, artificial, and skewed sample of behavior from which to draw conclusions.

Class and culture of both patient and therapist make a difference regarding diagnosis, prognosis, and treatment (Riessman, Cohen, & Pearl, 1964). When a patient is perceived as lower class (Hasse, 1964), he received a less favorable diagnosis than his middle-class counterpart, even when the case materials (e.g., Rorschach inkblot test protocols) are identical. Socioeconomic class also affects being accepted for services (Brill & Storrow, 1964), such that the lower the socioeconomic status, the lower the likelihood of being accepted for treatment; and once accepted for services, the treatment for the low-income individual is likely to be briefer, less intense, and given by a staff person with less status and experience (Hollingshead & Redlich, 1958). We are still seeing today the biases in diagnosis, prognosis, and treatment that were all too evident 100 years ago, embodied in the nineteenth century phrase "foreign insane pauperism" (Bockoven, 1956); we can guess at the class of the coiner of that phrase.

Ennis and Litwack (1974) conclude that "psychiatric judgments are not sufficiently reliable or valid to justify their admissibility under traditional rules of evidence," and recommend that "psychiatrists should not be permitted to testify as experts in civil commitment proceedings" (p. 735). They reinforce their point by analogy to the judicial treatment of polygraph results, which are not accepted in evidence by most courts; yet the polygraph, by conservative estimate, "can correctly detect truth or deception about 80 to 90 percent of the time" (p. 736). No psychiatric judgment can claim as much.

To quote Ennis and Litwack:

> The court gave five reasons for excluding lie detector results: (a) the possibility that extraneous qualities or characteristics of the subject might yield erroneous results; (b) the tendency of judges and juries to treat lie detector evidence as conclusive; (c) the lack of standardized testing procedures; (d) the difficulty of evaluating examiner opinions; and (e) the nonacceptance of the technique by appropriate scientific bodies.
>
> Each of these objections provides a cogent reason also to exclude psychiatric judgments: (a) extraneous qualities of psychiatric patients – such as their socioeconomic class – may substantially influence psychiatric judgments; (b) judges and juries usually defer to psychiatric judgments; (c) psychiatric interview procedures are unstandardized; (d) it is difficult for judges and juries to evaluate the validity of individual psychiatric judgments; and (e) psychiatrists and behavioral scientists almost unanimously agree that such judgments are of low reliability and validity. (p. 737)

The authors wish to limit psychiatrists in civil commitment hearings to descriptive statements only; diagnoses, opinions, and predictions would be inadmissible. It is clear that the legal and the mental health professions are questioning the latter's expertness and degree of certainty. For example, Ennis and Emery (1978) take issue with a justification for involuntary commitment and treatment put forward by Stone (1975); Stone suggested that forced treatment is justified because most mental patients who are treated involuntarily will be "thankful" for the treatment in hindsight. He believes that most patients would say "thank you for forcing treatment on me." Ennis and Emery (1978) disagree. So do I. That has not been my experience in working with patients who have been involuntarily confined and treated. Most resent deeply what happened, and carry their resentment for a long time, even to the point of souring current functioning.

The point is that whether someone will be "thankful" or not is an empirical question, impossible to predict ahead of time in individual cases. To use this justification is ". . . an unjustified and circular procedure, which, in practice, simply legitimizes the psychiatrist's opinion of what should be done" (Ennis & Emery, 1978, p. 42).

There are reasonable doubts regarding the validity of professional predictions. The doubts are so well founded and of such a serious nature that they are unquestionable. Yet within the realm of our doubt stands the alleged patient; and in some way, because of our doubt, his liberty is in greater jeopardy. We owe it to ourselves, our profession, the courts, and the alleged patient to "sort" our doubts, rather than to inflict them.

THE LEAST RESTRICTIVE ALTERNATIVE

Since no crime has been committed, should commitment and confinement be to an institution, such as a hospital, where the loss of freedom is great? This question has received fresh attention[20] as the court, mental health professional, legal advocate, family, and alleged patient grope for alternatives to hospitalization.

Confinement in a hospital has many drawbacks. Because state hospitals are often located away from populated areas, commitment not only involves relocation, but the breaking of existing community and neighborhood ties. It may mean the loss of a job and going from a financially secure to an insecure situation. It may mean the loss of an apartment and roommates. Contact with family and friends is likely to be reduced, if not severed. And whether treatment is really or rarely received, or is effective, are open questions. All of these shortcomings related to involuntary hospitalization make alternatives more attractive.

The Joint Commission on Mental Illness and Health Report (1961) identified state hospitals as our number-one mental health problem; this gave powerful impetus to the search for alternatives. That impetus is seen again in the 1978 Commission Report.

---

[20] *Eubanks* v. *Clarke* (1977). Reported in the *United States Law Week*, 1977, *46*, 3.

Community mental health centers, day hospitals, day treatment centers, half-way houses, residential homes, and group homes are some of the transitional facilities that have grown in response to the search for alternatives to the hospital.

The pressure is growing to use these alternatives. One reason stems from studies of hospital effectiveness. Anthony, Buell, Sharratt, and Althoff (1972) reviewed over 50 studies in which treatment took place in a hospital prior to discharge or on an outpatient basis. They used two criteria for judging effectiveness of treatment: recidivism (percentage of patients who return to the hospital) and post-hospital employment. Rappaport (1977) comments on this review and says, "If these criteria are accepted as the legitimate value/goals then it is clear that *in-hospital treatments, regardless of their nature and effectiveness at improving hospital behavior, do not differentially affect the discharged patient's community functioning.*" Thus "hospitalization may be, if not destructive, at least *irrelevant* to the ability of those with problems in living to learn to function in the real world" (p. 277).

From the same review of studies by Anthony and his associates comes evidence that aftercare follow-up counseling and autonomous alternative settings seem to be two promising alternatives to in-hospital treatment. Both aftercare and the use of a transitional facility (e.g., a half-way house) make better use of community, neighborhood, family, job, and social support systems than does hospitalization. On the basis of effectiveness, the less restrictive alternatives make good sense.

What does not make good sense, however, is to use these alternatives as part of *coercive* treatment. As Rappaport states in another section of his book (1977), "If the aim is treatment, in the sense of preparing a person for a useful role in society, then it will be necessary for treatment to be voluntary rather than forced" (p. 322). What this suggests is a different role for the judge and courts in nonemergency commitment hearings—that is, the bringing to bear of information regarding alternatives to hospitalization. I also think it is important, once the information (including pros and cons) about various treatment facilities is made known, to leave the choice of treatment modality to the alleged patient. Sometimes, and particularly in this current age when many are attempting to avoid involuntary in favor of voluntary commitment, the manifest choice hides latent coercion. A hypothetical example of this would be an alleged patient told he had the choice of outpatient treatment or living in a supervised group home, but also told that should he refuse both, he would be committed to a hospital. Obviously, the choice in this hypothetical example is not free of coercion.

The least restrictive alternative is one free of direct or insidious coercion of any degree. Looked at therapeutically, existing evidence tells us that truly voluntary treatment works best. If treatment is really the goal once the person is suspected of being "mentally ill" and "in need of treatment," and is brought before a nonemergency commitment hearing, then the choices ought to be presented to and left with the alleged patient – for him to decide. This may seem contradictory (i.e., supposing that the "mentally ill" can make a "rational" choice) or seem foolhardy (i.e., giving the choice, and hence the possibility of refusal of treatment, to the one "in need of treatment"), yet this is what I am advocating. Regarding "rational" choice, I am not sure very many voluntary patients seeking outpatient or private practice psychotherapy seek it for rational reasons; we know too much about unconscious motivations and neurotic reasons to assume "rationality." We do know, however, that making the voluntary commitment to therapy – that is, deciding on your own that you want it and then seeking it – is an important step and predictor of a favorable therapeutic outcome.

If we feel it is *foolhardy* to let the person decide, and perhaps refuse treatment, I would ask, in return, "But is it *dangerous?*" If what the person implies by "foolhardy" is that the person may injure someone or himself, then I would suggest that nonemergency commitment procedures (invoking *parens patriae*) are inappropriate, and that emergency procedures (invoking Mill's *harm* principle) should be instituted. I would hold however, to a rigorous definition of dangerous, which excludes danger to property, and requires evidence of threatened or attempted dangerous acts or an imminent threat of substantial physical harm. I would also further hold that the burden of proof falls on the one initiating emergency involuntary hospitalization.

If, however, foolhardy means silly or naive, or even insane, then I am willing to be all of those, rather than restricting someone's liberty on the basis of paternalistic presumption – that "father knows best" – when our empirical evidence reveals that we know precious little.

Looking legally at nonemergency involuntary hospitalization, if an alleged patient is given notice, has counsel, can cross-examine witnesses, challenge psychiatric diagnosis, avoid self-incrimination, and be subject to the proof beyond a reasonable doubt standard, then he stands a good chance of avoiding nonemergency commitment.

The nonemergency commitment, I think, is a failure on many levels. It seems to represent a virulent form of paternalism that leads to confinement in the name of treatment. A more cynical reader might say that it leads to confinement in lieu of treatment, if you read the right to treatment or effectiveness of hospitalization literature. I think this form of paternalism undermines *the possibility* of therapy. To make this point, we will review the basis of contractual therapy in the next section.

PATERNALISM IN CONTRACTUAL THERAPY

We have been dealing with the *involuntary* patient, how one gets to be such, and the problems, pitfalls, and paternalistic underpinnings that prop up, or threaten to pull down, such practices. We also started this major section with questions involving responsibility, and what happens when one avoids responsibility, and when another assumes it. In avoiding responsibility, the person was likened historically to the heretic, fool, blasphemer, madman, agent of the Devil, or Antichrist, to the physically sick, and the mentally ill. The painted likenesses have changed with the intellectual and moral climate of each age; compare the fifteenth century's image of madness as seen in Heironymus Bosch's *The Ship of Fools,* with the early twentieth century Picasso work *The Madman,* and we see the demonic giving way to the pathetic, evil yielding to pathos; yet, in both his diabolic and pathetic forms, a *child* has been seen.

The one who avoids responsibility has been and continues to be likened to a child. If responsibility is a good and necessary thing to have to insure responsible behavior, then significant others (e.g., friends, parents, spouse, teacher, police, courts, and mental health professionals) may take on the complimentary role of parent, to rear the child in the ways of responsibility and adult behavior. Thus the paternalistic dance begins.

At first blush it might be assumed that in contractual therapy — where two people come willingly to the dance — that paternalism, with its parent and child roles and coercive element, would not be a factor. Certainly, if we adhere strictly to the definition of paternalism given earlier, "Paternalism is the coercive interference with a person's liberty of action justified by reasons referring exclusively to the welfare, good, happiness, needs, interests, or values of the person being coerced," then we would be hard pressed to identify "clear, overt, or blatant" examples of coercion in voluntary contractual therapy. If we loosen our working definition, however, and acknowledge that both paternalism and coercion can come in various forms — sometimes covert, insidious, and unconscious – then a second or third look at psychotherapy might remove the blush of naivety. This is my proposal: to look at contractual therapy with an eye toward spotting paternalistic attitudes, roles, and actions, and comment on how it is handled therapeutically and ethically.

The theoretical literature on psychotherapy frequently invokes parent and child metaphors. The patient is pictured as childlike, dependent, regressed, and fixated, and therapy seeks to produce growth, autonomy, independence, and a healthy adult. In fact, therapy can be pictured as a process of transforming a child into an adult. The therapist as "transforming agent" may consciously play the parental role. Physicians have long been aware of the childishness that characterizes a sick person, as well as some of the added, placebo (psychological) benefits that result when the physician takes on the role of omnicompetent parent. As Menninger (1958) noted, "Some physicians almost consciously play the role of the grand father or the jocular uncle" (p. 78).

In the voluntary psychotherapeutic process, we not only have conscious attitudes and consciously assumed roles – but the *unconscious* as well. Freud (1953), in his 1912 paper entitled, "The Dynamics of Transference," pointed out that the patient will weave the figure of the physician into various roles or patterns already constructed in his mind. The physician may be woven into the image of a father, mother, sibling, employer, or others; and the patient's weaving, according to Freud, was unconscious, resulting primarily from the patient's neurosis, but, in part, from the analytic situation itself. Thus the therapist voluntarily becomes the parent when he consciously assumes that role, and involuntarily becomes the parent when the patient transfers the role onto him. There is a third way. The therapist may also become the parent out of his own unconscious dynamics – through countertransference. As Menninger states, "We may not forget that the psychoanalyst himself has an unconscious, and that he, too, has a persistent temptation to indulge in infantile techniques and objectives, magical thinking, and the like" (p. 84). He may have an unconscious need to be the parent, to "help" the patient in unnecessary ways, to offer premature reassurances, and to take charge in rearing the baby. If the transference and countertransference go on unrecognized and unchecked, we may wind up not rearing and transforming the child into an adult, but fostering and infantilizing the child. This therapeutic problem is quite similar to the parenting problem. How do you raise a child to become an adult? When do you do for the child and when does he do for himself? And when do you stop parenting and let go? Analogous paternalistic questions face the therapist. The following sections dealing with various stages of the therapeutic process, such as establishing a contract, handling the transference, and terminating therapy, illustrate the answers therapists give to these questions by their words and deeds.

THE THERAPEUTIC CONTRACT

The client comes to the therapist (in the usual circumstances) seeking "something." Talk ensues to find out what that "something" is, and whether it is appropriate and fitting with what the therapist is willing to offer; this may take one or several sessions (a precontractual period) to see if some agreement as to purpose (treatment goals) and logistics (time, money) can be reached. Therapy does not commence with a person's arrival at the office door. The prospective client may desire something the therapist is unwilling to give. If, for example, the prospective client perceives the world as threatening and unfulfilling, he may ask the therapist to protect and succor him. The therapist, if his general goal is to produce autonomy, independence, self-reliance and the like, may see the client's desire to have the therapist fulfill paternal and maternal needs as antithetical to growth. If this was the client's sole objective, the therapist may decline to take the case; or he may make a counter offer. The therapist might say, "I am not in the business of being a protective father or a nurturing mother, but I am in the business of helping people discover their own potentialities, such that they can protect and care for themselves." If this new goal sounds acceptable to the prospective client, a contract might be reached.

What can be seen through this illustration is that the therapist is sticking to his basic therapeutic goal of transforming, not fostering, the child. He begins this by not acceding to the client's childlike wish and role and by not taking on, for himself, the complimentary parental role. By evading the parental role, which would only place the client ever more securely in the child role, he opts for something that calls for more work and responsibility from the client. The therapist is seeking to ally himself with the "healthy ego" of the client, not the dependent, childlike, and neurotic side. Furthermore if the goal is to enlarge the healthy side, the process cannot begin by supporting the neurosis.

It should *not* be implied from the above example that the therapist *sets* the goals for the client, or determines what values the client should have, or how he ought to behave. It is not a one-way street — for that would be paternalism. The example does reveal that the therapist is a party to the process, that he has goals too, and that the therapeutic goals will have to be agreed to jointly. So values, goals, ethics, and morals, those of the client and the therapist, are important. If we accept Nicholas Hobbs' (1965) notion that "Psychotherapy may be described as an intimate dialogue about moral issues as lived by the client," then the therapist, by virtue of being "the party of the second part," is going to be immersed in a moralistic undertaking. The precontractual phase is (hopefully) to make clear the values and goals of both parties and to see if some common ground can be reached.

There are some who might disagree with the above assessment and claim instead that therapy is not a moralistic endeavor. If morals enter, they would assert that they enter as "slip-ups," improper technique, or countertransference feelings that should be corrected in supervision. This position, in the extreme, claims that the therapist (a) has no business becoming involved in the economic, political, moral, and religious beliefs of the client; (b) has no right to make value judgments of his client; (c) has no right to preach; and (d) should not dictate the "good" life for his client (London, 1964). This position sees therapy as analogous on the "tinkering trades" (Goffman, 1969) — those in the service guilds, like the watchmaker, TV repairman, and orthopedic surgeon, who provide a service like repairing one's watch, TV, or broken bones; in the main, these are not moralistic undertakings, and if there is as moral position here, it is Darwinian: that things ought to work as they were meant to work — so watches, TVs, and bones ought to be fixed.

The analogy between therapy and the tinkering trades, however, breaks down. We are, in therapy, not dealing with malfunctioning organs in the vast majority of cases. What we have instead are people whose thoughts and feelings are disturbed, and disturbed by still other thoughts and feelings. People seek treatment because of discrepancies between the way they see themselves and the way they want to be. Still others seek assistance for personal distress surrounding standards of conduct, human values, good and bad. As London (1964) has said, "much of the material he deals with is neither understandable nor usable outside the context of a system of human values. . . . Moral considerations may dictate, in large part, how the therapist defines his client's needs, how he operates in the therapeutic situation, how he defines 'treatment,' and 'cure,' and even 'reality'" (p. 5). London goes on to state that "the notion that the psychotherapist's situation differs much from the priest's is, I believe, a convenient fiction," and furthermore, calls the practitioners of psychotherapy "the secular priesthood" (p. 11).

Values, ethics, and morality are an integral part of therapy;

"that the very nature of his interaction with the people he serves involves a moral confrontation which, at the very least, renders communication of some part of his own moral commitments an inescapable part of his therapeutic work" (London, 1964, p. 11). The precontractual period is the time for making moral commitments clear. Again, to the extent that these matters are made clear and conscious, the less the likelihood of unconscious, paternalistic influences. The adverse effects of paternalism (i.e., the continuation of childhood and child–parent roles long past chronological maturity) may result from modeling and unconscious influences, as well as from conscious, paternalistic actions.

The essence of the psychotherapeutic contract, then, is openness and honesty; a balance has to be struck, and needs have to be reciprocally satisfied (Menninger, 1958). The best the therapist can do is to state honestly and openly his goals, beliefs, biases, and moral commitments. If the client likes what he hears and agrees to take his part in the dance, he has taken the first step toward growth — consciously assuming responsibility for himself. It is also the first step in therapeutically undoing the child–parent dichotomy.

TRANSFERENCE AND COUNTERTRANSFERENCE

In many forms of traditional psychotherapy — psychoanalysis and psychoanalytically oriented therapy being prime examples — the terms "transference" and "countertransference" are encountered, along with their respective manifestations. Freud felt that all of the patient's conflicts must be fought out on the field of transference for a proper cure to come about. Menninger (1958) quotes the words of Annie Reich that "countertransference is [not only an inevitable feature but also] a necessary prerequisite of analysis. If it does not exist, the necessary talent and interest is lacking" (p. 85). Thus transference and countertransference may be necessary ingredients for successful treatment. However, there are qualifiers that must be appended to this last sentence and safeguards placed on its practice. We will examine those qualifiers and safeguards shortly, but first some more on the nature and user of transference and countertransference.

Freud was amazed at the transference discovery. For him to be portrayed and reacted to "as if" he were someone else was baffling; what was most peculiar about the transference was its *excess,* in both *character* and *degree,* over what was rational and justifiable by the situation *per se.* So whereas he might understand a client treating him as her father, it was harder for him to understand her treating him as a lover—and it did not square with what he saw when he looked into the mirror. Yet, as therapy progressed and the patient regressed in order to progress, the transference "grew." One aspect of transference is the patient coming to see the therapist as a man who has the "magic word" and who could solve the problems and remove the patient's hurts with an oracular pronouncement. Yet the analyst remains silent. No pronouncements are forthcoming. In his frustration he may reenact childlike patterns and experiences to manipulate, control, seduce, or cajole an answer—still nothing. Why does the therapist not answer, or give the answer? First, because there is no answer—no answer that can come from "outside" or "on high" that magically produces change; and second, looking for the answer from the outside (from the therapist) diverts attention from the inside—from where the answer must come. So an external answer is not only no answer, it is worse. Giving external answers discourages looking within for internal answers. It discourages initiative and self-reliance. It infantilizes the client further. It promotes the very thing we are trying to undo—paternalism—in the form of a parent–child split.

Then what is the value of the regression and the developing transference? So the patient can see himself. See his methods and patterns of dealing with others. Witness his projections. If *he* sees it, the insights are *experienced* and *felt*. If he is told his patterns by the *therapist* who sees it, then the insights are the therapist's, and may not hit home for the client. Menninger's (1958) statement summarizes this point: "But the very spirit of psychoanalytic science is to help an afflicted ego to realize its *own* potentialities, to let a patient discover what he can really do—not because he is commanded to, not because it is diagrammed for him, but because he is acquiring a new view of himself" (p. 93).

As for countertransference, and, in particular, how it relates to paternalism, we can probably all see something of this sort going on within our own friendships and family relationships. We have needs to give, to nurture. These are usually beautiful, altruistic motives. Their expression may be just what our family and friends love about us and what makes us valuable friends. Yet giving, or giving to much or too quickly, can sometimes not be giving. Sometimes we give the best gift by not giving. Giving by not giving, sincerely wishing the best for the patient yet expressing an attitude of desirelessness, taking charge of treatment by letting the client take charge, being active by being passive, and providing insights by providing silence are some of the paradoxes of therapy. If the paradox is poorly resolved by the therapist, or worse, unnoticed, then the dangers of countertransference increase. The therapist may promote the child side of the client by promoting his own parent side.

The name of the game is for transference and countertransference to be seen, used, worked through, and then eliminated, so that each can see the other clearly, without distortions, fantasies, and projections getting in the way. The goal of the dance is for the client to discover the steps and recognize that he can lead, and ultimately, that he can dance alone.

TERMINATION OF THE CONTRACT

Termination is the concluding step, and a hard one. It is the "letting go" by both client and therapist of each other. When therapy goes on for 5, 10, or 20 years, one begins to wonder whether the partners desire to stop the dance. Is the dance interminable? Freud (1963) questioned this, in his 1937 paper entitled, "Analysis Terminable and Interminable." If analysis was ultimately education, or acquiring self-knowledge, is the lesson ever over? Perhaps not. Yet there may be a point to ending the twosome, and going it alone. This point often occurs, however, just when it gets "good" for both client and therapist: when distortions are gone, when a healthy sense of self has replaced a neurotic or childlike view of self, and when a true friendship seems within grasp. It may be difficult to let go.

Difficulties with letting go plague many parent–child relationships. There are strong desires to hang on, by both parties. Perhaps there are strong desires to turn the relationship into an adult friendship; many children have that wish as they grow older, yet find it difficult to do in practice. For in practice, the practice may have been exclusively as parent to child. It seems to me that the best examples of letting go and turning a parent–child relationship into an adult–adult relationship were those in which the "letting go" and "turning" started early – in the consciousness of the parents – who recognized from the beginning that the goal was ultimately to put themselves out of business. By gradually putting themselves out of the parenting business and role, they produce a corresponding role change and growth in the child turned adult. Psychological health and growth come when the child is reared and released, when the temporary assumption of responsibility has been gradually relinquished, and when the avoided responsibilities are reclaimed. So it seems with the therapeutic relationship.

Let us turn to involuntary confinement as treatment and see how these notions are played out there.

INVOLUNTARY CONFINEMENT AS TREATMENT

In 1955, the Congress of the United States passed the Mental Health Study Act which established a Joint Commission on Mental Health and Illness. The commission was to evaluate the current status of mental health services, pinpoint problems, and make recommendations regarding mental health needs, practices, and policies for the foreseeable future. In 1961, *Action for Mental Health: Final Report* (Joint Commission on Mental Illness and Health) was released. The report focused on three problem areas: (a) manpower, (b) facilities, and (c) costs; all three of these problem areas relate directly to the *major* problem facing the mental health movement—the chronic patient and his likely abode, the state mental hospital. As the report puts it, "major mental illness is the core problem and unfinished business of the mental health movement, and that the intensive treatment of patients with critical and prolonged mental breakdowns should have first call on fully trained members of the mental health professions" (p. xiv). Regarding state hospitals, the report recommends and concludes that "*Expenditures for public mental patient services should be doubled in the next five years—and tripled in the next ten.* Only by this magnitude of expenditure can typical state hospitals be made in fact what they are now in name only— hospitals for mental patients. . . . It is self-evident that the states, for the most part, have defaulted on adequate care for the mentally ill, and have consistently done so for a century."

My only "quibble" with this conclusion is that the default on adequate hospital care for the mentally ill, excluding a brief period of remission for moral treatment in the nineteenth century, has gone on for four centuries, or ever since hospitals or hôpitals got into the business of confining the mentally ill in the first place; and I feel that the Joint Commission Report of 1961 would likely read the same had it been released in 1861, 1761, or 1661.

History tempers us. It also teaches us. It leads us, by way of examples from each of the last four centuries, to anticipate our current failures that are voiced in the Joint Commission report. Perhaps history, or more properly, historiography, can awaken us to the reasons for our failures, and, by examining those historically brief successes we have enjoyed, remind us of "how to" and "how not to."

Turning the clock back, Foucault (1973) tells us that "Confinement was an institutional creation peculiar to the seventeenth century" (p. 63). The mentally ill, along with other "socially useless" individuals were confined, involuntarily for the most part, to Hôpitaux Généraux, houses of correction, and *Zuchthäusern* (work houses) to work. Foucault states that it did not work: "Measured by their functional value alone, the creation of the houses of confinement can be regarded as a failure" (p. 54). These houses did not work, nor did their inhabitants. Production and products, the outward, visible signs of work, failed to reach profitable levels; insight and awakening, the inward signs of work therapy, failed to materialize at any level. "In the workshops in which they were interned, they (the insane) distinguished themselves by their inability to work and to follow the rhythms of collective life" (Foucault, 1973, p. 58). Therapeutically, involuntary confinement was a failure, "a transitory and ineffectual remedy," "clumsily formulated" in the seventeenth century out of a fusion of industrial and ethical motives.

For 150 years, or from the founding of the Hôpital Général in 1656 to the end of the eighteenth century, the failure of confinement continued, grew worse, and, in general, receded from the consciousness of reasonable men. "Who thought about *those* places?" If these houses of confinement were given thought, or even visited, it was most likely because madmen made good spectacle; theatre, not therapy, became the thing that caught the consciousness of king and kin; 96,000 people a year visited the hospital of Bethlehem to witness and madman on display (Foucault, 1973).

When a serious eye was cast in the direction of hospitals — that is, of the late eighteenth and early nineteenth centuries — neglect, brutality, and fatality were the sights; *treatment* was nowhere to be found. At Bicêtre, the insane were in cells soaked by water. At La Salpêtriere, the waters and rats of the Seine filled dungeons. At the asylum of York, one room, less than 8 feet on a side, housed 13 women. At Bethlehem, there were chains from ankles to walls. At the hospital of Nantes, there were individual cages (Foucault, 1973). The attitude that pervaded was hopelessness. The patients got worse rather than better, with more dying than discharging occurring.

In the 1960s, when the Joint Commission and others (Goffman, 1961; Gruenberg, 1967; Zusman, 1973) looked at the state mental hospital, its practices and its patients, their assessment was not far different than the view in 1800. Patients got worse, in the main, not better, and what resulted was called a "social breakdown syndrome." As one writer has put it, "the hospitalized mentally ill respond to being crowded into locked, barred, unstimulating rooms by becoming deteriorated and animallike. Staff attitudes which give little hope for recovery, combined with the patients' not being permitted to wear their own clothing, have clocks, calendars, or mirrors, and an unchanging daily routine, lead to lack of concern for personal appearance, present activities, or future prospects. The social breakdown syndrome concept assumes a very direct relationship between the surroundings of a mentally ill person and the course of his illness" (Zusman, 1973, pp. 282–3).

As social breakdowns were occurring, discharges were not. The discharge figures, coupled with recidivism figures (those who return to the hospital following discharge), paint a bleak picture (Finkel, 1976). Looking at the discharge picture first, the probability of being discharged after spending 1 year in a hospital is 50%; the probability of being discharged after spending 2 years in a hospital drops to 20%; and the probability of being discharged after spending 5 years in a hospital sinks to 1%. Albee (1959) notes that 60% of the patients in state mental hospitals have been there over 5 years, and 40% of the patients have been there over 10 years. Chu and Trotter (1972) compare the length of stay figures for patients in St. Elizabeth's hospital with convicts in federal prisons. For the prisoner, 94% spend less than 5 years, 5% spend between 5 to 10 years, and 1% spend 10 to 40-plus years there. For patients in St. Elizabeth's, 34% spend less than 5 years, 13% spend 5 to 10 years, 16% spend 10 to 19 years, 29% spend 20 to 39 years, and 8% spend more than 40 years there. So in all but the short-term category (less than 5 years), patients are likely to spend more time in their facility than prisoners are in theirs.

As the length of stay increases, the average age of the patients increases, and psychiatric wards come to resemble geriatric wards (Goldhamer & Marshall, 1949); the results for the psychiatric and geriatric patient come to be identical—they stand a good chance of spending their last days of this world in the netherworld of the hospital.

When we add the recidivism figures to the picture, the light on the subject dims even further. The base rates for recidivism 1 year after hospitalization are from 30% to 50% (Rappaport, 1977); the probability of release from the hospital and stay in the community following 2 years of continuous hospitalization is about 6% (Paul, 1969), and this figure has been remarkably constant for a century.

As a *treatment* facility, the Hôpital Général, madhouse, asylum, or psychiatric hospital (call it what you will) cannot be called anything but a "failure." It arose as an institution of confinement; it has done that, but little else. In the seventeenth and eighteenth centuries, these houses of confinement served as ethical and moral punishment; in the nineteenth century, psychiatric hospitals replaced asylums in name and number, and "treatment" replaced "punishment" as the reason for confinement; yet from our twentieth century perspective, we see that the "grand experiment" has failed—"treatment" and patients have not emerged from those houses of confinement. The psychiatric hospital—the proposed solution—has become the problem (Finkel, 1976).

What we do see is the institution and the patient contributing to produce an *institutionalization syndrome:* the patient, for his part, demonstrates little responsibility and much childlike, dependent behavior; the institution, for its part, assumes most of decision-making responsibility, deciding when patients will eat, sleep, medicate, take recreation, receive passes, and be allowed privileges.

Goffman (1973) says that the chronic mental patient has chosen the patient role as a *moral career:* he comes to accept his new image as a patient, victim, sufferer, and loser. Braginsky, Braginsky, and Ring (1969) echo Goffman's notions: "First, we have argued that in a certain sense an individual *chooses* his career as a mental patient; it is not thrust upon him as a consequence of his somehow becoming 'mentally ill.' . . . Furthermore, given the life circumstances of most of the persons who become and remain residents of mental hospitals, their doing so evinces a realistic appraisal of their available alternatives; it is, in short, a rational choice" (p. 171). Braginsky, Grosse, and Ring (1973) demonstrated that patients engage in impression management as a manipulative tactic for getting what they want: the old timers worked for what they wanted, staying in the hospital, by presenting themselves as "ill" as measured by a mental illness test; the short timers worked for what they wanted, discharge, by presenting themselves as "insightful" on a self-insight test. Braginsky and Braginsky (1973) have demonstrated impression management in long-term schizophrenic patients in a psychiatric interview situation, where the desired end was living on an open ward. These studies point to a view of the patient as a more active and effective organism than one might have first thought, yet he acts, affects, and chooses to continue his career as a mental patient, rather than seek treatment and discharge. In short, given a chronic patient, he works to remain such and typically, the hospital aids in that process. Could the paternalistic–infantilistic bond be any securer, as both patient and hospital work toward "the making of a mental patient" (Price & Denner, 1973)?

What is the typical outcome? Patients do not come out from either hospitals or their career. So we are left with confinement in lieu of treatment, or, as the Joint Commission report put it, hospitals "in name only."

A RIGHT TO TREATMENT

The courts, however, through involuntary commitment proceedings, commit patients to hospitals *for treatment*. We begin to see the problem and the contradiction. Commitment for the purpose of treatment, yet the promise of treatment is unfulfilled. These facts have prompted a number of "right to treatment" cases, the most prominent of which are *Donaldson* v. *O'Connor* and *Wyatt* v. *Stickney*. Before we proceed with the details and issues the cases raise, let us pause to take in the *irony*: we have patients involuntarily committed to hospitals for treatment arguing that they are not getting it. "Not getting treatment in a hospital, you say. Then what are they getting?"

Kenneth Donaldson, after telling his father that someone, perhaps a neighbor, might be putting something in his food (Ennis, 1972), underwent a sanity hearing, was given a diagnosis of "paranoid schizophrenia," and then spent the next 15 years in Florida State Hospital. His documented complaints to the Florida legislature described his building as "antiquated," "completely obsolete," and "a serious fire hazard." The following passage gives an account of what it was like (Ennis, 1972):

> The wards were "maintained more as detention wards for inmates than as hospital wards for the sick." It was a "common practice" for attendants to "choke" agitated patients until they were subdued. The committee discovered "strip cells," where patients were held naked in solitary confinement, without bedding or exercise, for "prolonged" periods. Attendants, not doctors, decided which patients would be put there and for how long. A "large number" of those attendants had "less than a high school education" and were "ill-equipped for the responsible care and treatment of patients." The average take-home pay for attendants was less than $1,700 per year. Forced to moonlight in order to survive, the attendants

frequently were too exhausted to give patients the attention they required and considered their duties "almost exclusively custodial in nature."

The hospital, in general, was "extremely short of doctors," the report continued, but the shortage was most acute in Donaldson's section, where "during 1960 and prior to that time, there was only one doctor [an obstetrician] responsible for the care and treatment of approximately 1,000 [male] patients" (the American Psychiatric Association considered one doctor for every 150 patients to be the absolute minimum). There was no psychiatrist, no psychologist, and, except in the infirmary, no nurse. It was not uncommon for patients to go two, three, or even four years without speaking to a doctor. (pp. 105–106)

That was Donaldson's *treatment*.

Ricky Wyatt, a patient in Bryce Hospital in Alabama, did not fare much better. The brief of *Amici Curiae* filed in the United States Court of Appeals for the Fifth Circuit, documented over-crowding, inadequate plumbing, little or no privacy, health haz-ards, and a lack of safety. A nutritional expert testified "that malnutrition could be a causal factor of inmate mental problems, and that adequate nutrition was an important element of treat-ment." Furthermore, it was admitted that "somewhat less than 50 cents per patient a day" was allotted for food. This amounts to $3.50 per week. Bockoven (1956) cites figures for the year 1869, where, at Worcester State Hospital, the weekly cost per patient was $4.00, as was the per capita income of the United States. In 1899, when the per capita income of the United States rose to $5.00 per week, the weekly cost per patient at Worcester had dropped to $3.50 per week. In 1971, when the Wyatt case was working its way through the courts, patients were being fed on $3.50 per week.

In addition, there were accounts of exploitive patient labor, misuses of solitary confinement and restraints, and brutality and inmate deaths. Regarding staffing, there was one medical doctor with some psychiatric training for 5000 inmates, one Ph.D. psy-chologist for every 1670 inmates, and one masters-level social worker for every 2500 inmates; and last, there seemed to be no individualized treatment plan for inmates.

Judge Johnson, ruling in the Wyatt (Note 11) case, wrote as follows:

The patients at Bryce Hospital, for the most part, were involuntar-ily committed through noncriminal proceedings and without the constitutional protections that are afforded defendants in criminal proceedings. When patients are so committed for treatment purposes they unquestionably have a constitutional right to receive such individual treatment as will give each of them a realistic opportunity to be cured or to improve his or her mental condition. (p. 784)

Judge Johnson seemed to be following the lead of Judge Bazelon, an acknowledged judicial expert in mental health law, who had written, "If the legislative promise of treatment is dishonored, involuntary and indefinite 'hospitalization' amounts to no more than preventive detention" (Bazelon, 1969, p. 2).

When the Supreme Court heard the Donaldson case,[21] they were not impressed by the "treatment" he received. The following section comes from Mr. Justice Stewart's opinion: "O'Connor described Donaldson's treatment as 'milieu therapy.' But witnesses from the hospital staff conceded that, in the context of this case, 'milieu therapy' was a euphemism for confinement in the 'milieu' of a mental hospital."

As the courts have begun to move toward the acknowledgement of a "right to treatment," their movement has, in turn, caused a resonating movement within state legislatures, hospitals, and among hospital patients and doctors. State legislatures are confronted with much larger budgets for mental hospitals if they are to "be made in fact what they are now in name only — hospitals for mental patients." This means repair, renovation, and hiring of new staff; a large expense in an age of tight budgets. Hospitals seem to be moving, in reaction to right to treatment suits, toward quicker, and, sometimes, mass release of patients as a way of (a) avoiding class action suits, (b) lowering patient-to-staff ratios to less objectionable levels, and (c) lowering their budgets to more justifiable levels. As a result, patients are moving out, in great numbers, back to their communities; however, both the community and the patient may be ill prepared for such an adventure. Such is the case as told by Peter Koenig (*The New York Times Magazine,* May 21, 1978), in an article entitled, "The Problem That Can't Be Tranquilized," with a subheading, "40,000 Mental Patients Dumped in City Neighborhoods": this article describes the new syndrome of "dumping" — and its effects on patients, neighborhoods, and communities. The article describes the quick release of patients, with the lack of aftercare planning and follow-through in many cases, along with the living arrangements and single-room occupant (SRO) — flop houses — which come to house the dumped. Neighborhoods are beginning to complain about these "social marginals": a former head of a

---

[21] *O'Connor* v. *Donaldson,* 422 U. S. 563 (1975).

local community board was quoted as saying, "We feel on the Upper West Side that we have as many social marginals as we can deal with. We can't take any more." Shades of Foucault! The complaints sound like those of the good residents of Paris in the sixteenth century, who also feared being overrun by madness.

The dumped often become victims of crime (e.g., robbery, burglary, assaults, murder). As Lieutenant D. Velez states, "In most cases, the mentally disabled are victims of crime, not perpetrators, especially if they live in SROs. You're throwing goldfish among the piranhas there." Yet our psychological literature tells us that victims are often blamed, rather than sympathized with, for their plight. Just by being there, by being easy targets, they contribute to "the general chaos" of a neighborhood feeling itself on the edge of Thanatos. When this happens, and frustration mounts, people begin to "confuse their fear of crime with their fear of insanity." In the same month and year (this time, *Newsweek*, May 8, 1978), an article entitled, "Insanity on Trial," appeared in the popular press. It concerned, in part, communities' fears that the insanity defense was" little more than a ploy used by killers, abetted by crafty defense lawyers and soft-hearted psychiatrists, to escape punishment." The article also dealt with the communities' confusion of criminality and mental illness, and fears that the mentally ill are dangerous (see previous section on predictions of dangerousness), and ought to be securely (and permanently?) locked up. Whether a community looks at the mentally ill with fear or compassion, whether it welcomes them back or shuns them, depends on "the collective feeling of security within a community." Community sentiment today seems ambivalent: there is shock at stories of hospital back wards being snakepits, but worry about the snakepit moving into their own backyard.

What has resulted, at the patient–community nexus, is a "revolving-door syndrome," where the chronically ill are first hospitalized, then dumped, then readmitted, and then dumped again.

The hospital physician, besides signing discharge and re-admittance slips at a dizzy rate, is increasingly finding himself caught in the middle of the revolving door: formerly he was charged and sued for not doing enough and not releasing patients quickly enough, but, in more recent days, suits are being brought claiming that doctors are releasing patients too quickly. Having gotten himself into the paternal role of assuming responsibility, he finds himself facing suits from both directions. An insane position to be caught in, one might say.

MORAL TREATMENT

Hospitals have begun to reexamine their practices, and institute change. The 1960s produced renewed interest in the state mental hospital, and several newer treatment approaches made their debut. A large impetus for these new approaches no doubt came from the Joint Commission report. Yet change, particularly hospital change, does not come easily, since "the hospital has not always been hospitable to change" (Finkel, 1976, p. 83). As Rappaport, Chinsky, and Cowen (1971) write, "In many ways, the challenge of introducing significant change into a state hospital can be likened to the problem of awakening a sleeping dragon — one on a continuous dose of thorazine!" (p. 40). One discovery that has been made in the search for *new* treatments is the rediscovery of an *old* treatment — moral treatment — which Bockoven called psychiatry's "forgotten success."

Bockoven (1956) defines moral treatment in the following passage:

> Humanitarianism favored the view that lunatics had undergone stresses which robbed them of their reason. That such stress could result from disappointment as well as inflammation was a basic assumption. Stresses of a psychological nature were referred to as *moral causes.* Treatment was called *moral treatment,* which meant that the patient was made comfortable, his interest aroused, his friendship invited, and discussion of his troubles encouraged. His time was managed and filled with purposeful activity. (p. 178)

The goal of this emotional or psychological treatment approach, in the words of Samuel Tuke, grandson of William Tuke who founded the Retreat near York, was "to awaken the slumbering reason" (Tuke, 1813, p. 23). This goal was to be accomplished without resort to the physical accoutrements of confinement, bars, chains, and restraints. Patients, in England, at Tuke's Quaker Retreat, and in France, at Pinel's Bicêtre, were being liberated from the physical restraints. Foucault describes the liberation in France in the following passage (1973):

> As for the liberation of the insane at Bicêtre, the story is famous: the decision to remove the chains from the prisoners in the dungeons; Couthon visiting the hospital to find out whether any suspects were being hidden; Pinel courageously going to meet him, while everyone trembled at the sight of the "invalid carried in men's arms." The confrontation of the wise, firm philanthropist and the paralytic monster. "Pinel immediately led him to the section for the deranged, where the sight of the cells made a painful

impression on him. He asked to interrogate all the patients. From most, he received only insults and obscene apostrophes. It was useless to prolong the interview. Turning to Pinel: 'Now, citizen, are you mad yourself to seek to unchain such beasts?' Pinel replied calmly: "Citizen, I am convinced that these madmen are so intractable only because they have been deprived of air and liberty."

" 'Well, do as you like with them, but I fear you may become the victim of your own presumption." Whereupon, Couthon was taken to his carriage. His departure was a relief; everyone breathed again; the great philanthropist immediately set to work." (p. 242)

What was happening was that the old notions of punishment, dangerousness, and safety were giving way to treatment, humanism, and voluntarism. Tuke (1813) wrote about these changes from the old to the new in the following passage:

> Many errors in the construction, as well as in the management of asylums for the insane, appear to arise from excessive attention to *safety*. People, in general, have the most erroneous notions of the constantly outrageous behaviour, or malicious dispositions, of deranged persons; and it has, in too many instances, been found convenient to encourage these false sentiments, to apologize for the treatment of the unhappy sufferers, or admit the vicious neglect of their attendants.
>
> In the construction of such places, cure and comfort ought to be as much considered, as security; and, I have no hesitation in declaring, that a system which, by limiting the power of the attendant, obliges him not to neglect his duty, and makes it his interest to obtain the good opinion of those under his care, provides more effectually for the safety of the keeper, as well as of the patient, than all "the apparatus of chains, darkness, and anodynes." (pp. 106–107)

As moral therapists were creating "communities" of hope, spirit, and confidence where education, meaningful work, and psychological insight could come about through the law of love, they were achieving success rates unmatched in history. The Retreat gave figures (Tuke, 1813) showing that 84% of their recent cases of mania and melancholic disorders were cured or much improved. In the United States, the Hartford Retreat reported 90% recovery figures using moral treatment, although the population had less than one year of hospitalization. At Worcester State Hospital, a facility also using moral treatment, the discharged as recovered or improved figure was 71% during the 1833 –1842 period (Bockoven, 1956).

When we examine twentieth century hospital changes, we cannot help but "see" and "hear" the ghosts and echoes of moral treatment. Sullivan, in 1930, working with schizophrenics, proposed a therapeutic environment where the mental hospital would become a school for "personality growth rather than a custodian of personality failures" (Zusman, 1973). The British experiment of open hospitals following World War II took as its guiding principle the notion that mental patients are able to assume much more responsibility for themselves than many believed possible—another moral treatment assumption. Fairweather (1964), Sanders (1967), and Towbin (1969) all experimented with smaller units (e.g., cottages, lodges, separate wards) to create a community-at-large atmosphere. Maxwell Jones' (1953) notion of a therapeutic community is a direct descendent of Pinel's moral therapy. Rubenstein and Lasswell's (1966) book, interestingly entitled *The Sharing of Power in a Psychiatric Hospital,* discusses the patient as participant in his own cure as a new goal of treatment, and patient government is one way of aiding in the realization of that goal. The use of student volunteers and the creation of student-companion programs (Holzberg, Whiting, & Lowy, 1969; Poser, 1966; Rappaport, Chinsky, & Cowen, 1971; Umbarger, Dalsimer, Morrison, & Breggin, 1962) bring to the hospital "generalized enthusiasm," hope, and more interpersonal interactions—goals quite consistent with those of moral treatment.

If there is a theme to these successes, past and present, it could be capsulized in the following way: paternalism needs to be undone. When wards are opened rather than closed, when responsibilities are given and shared rather than taken and assumed, and when treatment is provided and voluntarily sought rather than involuntarily administered, patients get better rather than more chronic and exit rather than stay.

Involuntary confinement has not proved to be treatment; in fact, its effects and practices become indiscriminable from punishment; its results worse. Paternalism, the underlying ideology beneath involuntary confinement, can only be judged as a therapeutic failure. The patient does not grow up. The moral, here, is obvious.

4

CONTROL, RESPONSIBILITY, FREEDOM, AND DIGNITY

There is a case for control. It would not be stated or argued for by a traditional, insight-oriented therapist, though; it would be made by the action-oriented therapist (London, 1964). The "actionist," as London coins this breed of man, is different than his brother, the insight-oriented therapist; for he grew up and grew comfortable with "behavioristic psychotherapists" or "learning theory based psychotherapists," rather than traditional *fare au Freud et al.*; and as a result, he *saw* a little differently. He saw that, "To state the obvious, we are all in the business of control" (Goldfried & Davison, 1976, p. 267). His therapeutic philosophy and purpose is behavior change, not insight; for insights could be profound and wonderous, textured and colorful, and layered with symbols and sequins one atop another — without a stitch changing. If behavior change is the prime therapeutic goal, as the actionist argues it should be, then firm and effective control should be sought, not avoided. If any aversive aftertaste or queasiness to taking control remains, as well it might following traditional therapeutic fare, digestion will be more than compensated for by therapeutic results.

The portrait of the actionist is done in "bolder" and "rudder" lines (London, 1964). Contrary to the grey and subdued colors of the insight therapist, who watches, guides, counsels, and Socratizes (Skinner, 1971) his clients, and who exerts discretion, circumspection, and as little control as possible save on controlling

88

The Case for Controls versus the Right to Refuse Treatment

and checking himself in guiding his client through the straits of Scylla, Charybdis, Jackets and Life ("a local law firm"), the actionist will use intense control, if he has to, be it argument, seduction, threat, or skillful violence (à la the surgeon) to excise the symptom and change the behavior. For "behavior change" is the name of his game; and if this calls for "a momentary autocracy," then "So be it!," says the actionist.

This portrait of the actionist may be unfair, lopsided, and unflattering as caricatures tend to be, with one or two features exaggerated while the rest are blurred or omitted. One frequent caricature of the actionist is as a Machiavellian schemer, shrewdly manipulating variables and people at the cost of dignity and freedom. It may be that the artist's (and our own) "sense of autonomy" and "free will" seem jeopardized, so we project and paint the actionist in darker, more sinister tones. The actionist, in his own defense and best therapeutic manner, would no doubt comfort us: "Fear not," he might say; "You have nothing to fear from me. I can not take from you what you never had. Your 'free will' and the little 'autonomous man' within you, those two comforting though ineffective constructs (illusions) are safe. I leave illusions, introspective voyages, and 'sleight of mind' tricks to my therapeutic brother, the insight-oriented therapist. I do not manipulate illusions. Only behavior."

Whether the reader is properly comforted or not, it is time to move from caricature and hypothetical dialogue to B.F. Skinner, the titular head of the behaviorist perspective, and his thoughts on change, control, freedom, responsibility, and the like. The following quotes and points are taken from his provocative work, *Beyond Freedom and Dignity* (1971).

Skinner raises the question, where, or with whom, does responsibility lie in the control of behavior and its changing? He tells us that the traditional view has placed responsibility within the organism, as a function of man's autonomous being and his free will. Skinner's own view, in contrast, is predicated on determinism and grounded in a scientific method, which "shifts both the responsibility and the achievement to the environment" (p. 23). Not only does responsibility change in its locus, for Skinner it now takes a back seat to control, as the following quoted passage reveals:

> The real issue is the effectiveness of techniques of control. We shall not solve the problems of alcoholism and juvenile delinquency by increasing a sense of responsibility. It is the environment which is "responsible" for the objectionable behavior, and it is the environment, not some attribute of the individual, which must be changed. . . . The concept of responsibility offers little help. The issue is controllability. . . . What must be changed is not the responsibility of autonomous man but the conditions, environmental or genetic, of which a person's behavior is a function. (pp. 70–71)

Skinner reviews the therapeutic strategies of those "who champion freedom and dignity; he covers permissiveness, midwifery (Socratic technique of drawing the truth out), guidance, and changing minds. His general conclusion is that, "Their (those who champion freedom and dignity) concern for autonomous man commits them to only ineffective measures" (p. 78).

Specifically, "Permissiveness is not, however, a policy; it is the abandonment of policy, and its apparent advantages are illusory. To refuse to control is to leave control not to the person himself, but to other parts of the social and nonsocial environments" (p. 79).

Skinner characterizes the midwife metaphor in the following way: "The patient is not to be told how to behave more effectively or given directions for solving his problems; a solution is already within him and has only to be drawn out with the help of the midwife–therapist." Skinner sees midwifery as more effective than permissiveness, probably achieving results, when it does achieve results, precisely because more control is exerted. The midwife-practitioner, however, in Skinner's judgment, "avoids responsibility. Just as it is not the midwife's fault if the baby is stillborn or deformed, so the teacher is exonerated when the student fails, the psycho-therapist when the patient does not solve his problems, and the mystical religious leader when his disciples behave badly" (p. 81).

Guidance and changing minds fare just as poorly, in Skinner's estimation. "Guidance is effective, however, only to the extent that control is exerted. To guide is either to open new opportunities or to block growth in particular directions. To arrange an opportunity is not a very positive act, but it is nevertheless a form of control if it increases the likelihood that behavior will be emitted. The teacher who merely selects the material the student is to study or the therapist who merely suggests a different job or change of scene has exerted control, though it may be hard to detect" (p. 83). Yet guidance ducks the responsibility issue, since "one who merely guides is exonerated when things go wrong" (p. 82).

Skinner's sharpest words are saved for the mind changers. He writes:

> It is a surprising fact that those who object most violently to the manipulation of behavior nevertheless make the most vigorous efforts to manipulate minds. Evidently freedom and dignity are threatened only when behavior is changed by physically changing the environment. There appears to be no threat when the states of mind said to be responsible for behavior are changed, presumably because autonomous man possesses miraculous powers which enable him to yield or resist.
>
> It is fortunate that those who object to the manipulation of behavior feel free to manipulate minds, since otherwise they would have to remain silent. But no one directly changes a mind. By manipulating environmental contingencies, one makes changes which are said to indicate a change of mind, but if there is any effect, it is on behavior. The control is inconspicuous and not very effective, and some control therefore seems to be retained by the person whose mind changes. (Skinner, 1971, pp. 86–87)

What we are left with, as Skinner sees it, when "apparent freedom" is respected by weak therapeutic measures, "is merely inconspicuous control" (p. 92), which yields ineffective therapy.

Another behaviorally oriented therapist, Albert Bandura (1969), sounds a similar note to Skinner in contrasting traditional conversational therapy with behavioral therapy:

> Psychotherapists who subscribe to conversational methods customarily portray their form of treatment as a noncontigent social influence process in which the therapist serves as an unconditionally loving, permissive, understanding, empathizing catalyst in the client's efforts toward self-discovery and self-actualization. In contrast, behaviorally oriented psychotherapists are typically depicted

an antihumanistic, Machiavellian manipulators of human behavior. . . . In truth, to the extent that the psychotherapist — regardless of his theoretical allegiances — has been successful in modifying his client's behavior, he has either deliberately or unwittingly manipulated the factors that control it. It is interesting to note in this connection that conditions that are undesignedly imposed upon others are generally regarded with favor, whereas identical conditions created after thoughtful consideration of their effects on others are often considered culpable. There exists no other enterprise which values incognizance so highly, often at the expense of the client's welfare. (Bandura, 1969, p. 81)

Skinner picks up Bandura's point regarding "incognizance" as opposed to a planned, controlled intervention. His summary and concluding comments are worth quoting as a conclusion to this section.

The fundamental mistake made by all those who choose weak methods of control is to assume that the balance of control is left to the individual, when in fact it is left to other conditions. . . . The freedom and dignity of autonomous man seem to be preserved when only weak forms of nonaversive control are used. Those who use them seem to defend themselves against the charge that they are attempting to control behavior, and they are exonerated when things go wrong. Permissiveness is the absence of control, and if it appears to lead to desirable results, it is only because of other contingencies. Maieutics, or the art of midwifery, seems to leave behavior to be credited to those who give birth to it, and the guidance of development to those who develop. . . . Various ways of changing behavior by changing minds are not only condoned but vigorously practiced by the defenders of freedom and dignity. There is a good deal to be said for minimizing current control by other people, but other measures still operate. A person who responds in acceptable ways to weak forms of control may have been changed by contingencies which are no longer operative. By refusing to recognize them the defenders of freedom and dignity encourage the misuse of controlling practices and block progress toward a more effective technology of behavior. (Skinner, 1971, pp. 94–95)

THE ACTIONIST'S
"CRITIQUE OF PURE INSIGHT"

Philosophical, theoretical, and technical differences split the action and insight-oriented therapists. Dichotomies such as freedom versus determinism, humanism versus mechanism, and self-knowledge versus symptom change have characterized the split and difference of focus between these two orientations. The split was occurring in Freud's day, and in his own treatment approach, when he began to shift from hypnosis to the newly emerging psychoanalytic method. In the older, hypnotic method, the doctor was active, doing much of the talking and all of the leading and directing; in short, he was in charge of the treatment and responsible for its outcome. When Freud shifted to the psychoanalytic method of free association, the doctor grew silent, listening rather than talking, following rather than leading; in short, it was the patient who knew (at least, unconsciously knew) where the conflicts were, and it was he who had to take the lead and responsibility in getting to them.

To someone like Skinner, Freud's change of method seems confusing and inconsistent; Freud the determinist, that tough-nosed scientist who tried to put psychology on a scientific footing,[1] was seemingly shifting to give the patient "freedom" and free will to lead his own treatment, uncover unconscious causes, and undo symptoms. Skinner (1971) focused on the determinist-free will inconsistency when he wrote "Freud was a determinist — on faith, if not on the evidence — but many Freudians have no hesitation in assuring their patients that they are free to choose among different courses of action and are in the long run the architects of their own destinies" (p. 18).

More than a philosophical confusion between determinism and free will riles Skinner and the actionists. As they see it, letting the responsibility for the therapeutic mission's success rest with the patient — who has neither a conscious understanding of his condition, nor a therapeutic plan — is folly. As London (1964) states, "Action therapists would no more ask their patients to conduct their own treatment than doctors would ask patients to prescribe their own medicines" (pp. 78–79). The actionist asks his insight brethren some tough, pointed questions: "Isn't giving responsibility to the patient like having the blind leading the guide dog, or letting the child strike matches while the parent fiddles?" "Is *assuming* that the patient can assume responsibility just a cloak for a therapist *avoiding* his responsibility to lead, guide, and control the therapeutic mission?"

The actionist comes to the question of therapeutic control with an empirical bent. What has history taught us regarding what works and what does not? As Thoresen and Mahoney (1974) state, "Many things, of course, are simply not within our power to control, but many more are than is generally conceded by layman and professional alike. Epictetus, the ancient Stoic philosopher,

---

[1] See Freud (1974), Project for a Scientific Psychology (1895).

observed almost 2000 years ago that human actions — thoughts, emotions, opinions, aversions — were within a person's power to control, if he *believed* in such a possibility . . . (pp. vii, viii).

Despite the wisdom of Epictetus and others, we have remained essentially ignorant of *how* to control our own acts. Admonishments to "know thyself," to exert willpower, or to think positively have not sufficed (pp. vii–viii). So throwing the responsibility and burden of therapy onto the patient and his "willpower," "free will," "consciousness," "self-direction," "soul," "personality," or "self-knowledge" may be a case of invoking therapeutically empty constructs that neither speak nor function. The actionist sees the insight therapist giving the patient *choice* and *control*, whereas the actionist assigns both to the therapist (London, 1964). London cites two actionists, Wolpe and Skinner, regarding the responsibility for choice and control, "Wolpe does not hesitate to take responsibility for his decisions, and the Skinnerian position does not allow the possibility even that responsibility could rest anywhere else than with the therapist" (p. 120).

As a concluding thought on this section, a quotation from London's chapter, "An Epitaph For Insight," is offered:

> That the locus of control in therapy should reside in the therapist rather than the patient may seem reprehensible to some people who are accustomed to one or another Insight model of psychotherapy. But the Actionist may fairly claim, from within the framework of his assumptions, that he is doing much the same thing a physician does in the treatment of a symptom of physical illness. Viewed that way, the most reprehensible behavior of which the Action therapist can be accused is that he uses his own judgment in the conduct of the treatment. The outcome of his treatment may radically alter the life of the patient, but that is no argument one way or the other for attempting it. Surgery radically alters people's lives, and so can the recommendation that they move to another climate, take exercise, or stop smoking. It is perhaps less presumptuous of the doctor, when all is said and done, to treat the symptom with some disdain for its role in the total life of the patient, than to think too far ahead of its consequences. (London, 1964, pp. 120–121)

CONTROLS, VALUES, AND CONSENT

Control, particularly effective control, is a force that upsets inertia, alters current courses, and moves objects, people, and behaviors from one place or state to another. Like physical forces, psychological forces have a directional component too: we have *goals*. Goals, however, are a different order of reality from controls and forces, and pose different questions: where controls deal in technology – "a how to" language – so to speak, goals deal with targets and who sets them and why: the question of values.

It is here, usually, that the insight-oriented therapist seizes the offensive and sees equivocation at best and paternalism at worst in the values and actions of his actionist brethren. London (1964) tells us that, by and large, the actionist selects the goals of therapy:

> Just as the Action therapist is deliberately responsible for the conduct of treatment, he tends to be responsible in large part for its outcome too; he tends, in other words, to select in advance the particular changes he wishes to effect in the behavior of his patient. . . . Even if he gives his patient a choice of goals, as doctors sometimes do, he himself defines what goals are possible; Insight therapists, contrarily, leave the onus of defining treatment goals on the patient to begin with. (pp. 79–80)

The "equivocation" is seen when we examine the words of another behaviorally oriented therapist, Bandura, who takes a different position from that which London claims for the actionist. Bandura (1969) separates the decision of selection of goals from the technical procedures for achieving goals, and argues that the client must be the chief decision maker for the former, the therapist, for the latter. He states:

> In any type of social influence enterprise there exist two basic decision systems. One set of decisions pertains to the selection of goals; these decisions require value judgments. The second set of decisions, which involve empirical issues, relates to the selection of specific procedures for achieving selected goals. In the latter domain the agent of change must be the decision-maker, since the client is in no position to prescribe the learning contingencies necessary for the modification of his behavior. But though the change agent determines the means by which specified outcomes can be achieved, the client should play a major role in determining the directions in which his behavior is to be modified. To the extent that the client serves as the primary decision-maker in the value domain, the ethical questions that are frequently raised concerning behavioral control become pseudo issues. (Bandura, 1969, p. 101)

Bandura is certainly trying to put distance between his own brand of behavioral therapy and the caricatured Machiavellian schemer who rides rough shod over value concerns. He writes,

"Moreover, ethical considerations require that clients specify the ways in which they wish to be changed, that the intended outcomes of the therapeutic process be made known, and that clients be informed of the likelihood that the treatment interventions will enable them to deal more effectively with the life problems for which they seek help" (p. 60).

But Bandura is not out of the woods yet. Although a *paper* distinction between values and goals, on the one hand, and empirical techniques on the other may be clear, *in practice* things get quite blurry. Clients seldom come into therapy with clearly stated goals in mind. Typically, their goals (if they are stated at all) are stated too vaguely, broadly, and wistfully; certainly not behaviorally. How, then, does the therapist translate ephemeral yearnings into practical tasks? Conversation between therapist and client ensues to "sharpen" and operationalize goals. However neutral the therapist wishes to remain, however much he wishes the client to state his own goals and for himself to stay out of this decision, most agree that "therapeutic neutrality" is a myth (Bandura, 1969; Goldfried & Davison, 1976; Halleck 1971). As Halleck states:

> At first glance, a model of psychiatric practice based on the contention that people should just be helped to learn to do the things they want to do seems uncomplicated and desirable. But it is an unobtainable model. Unlike a technician, a psychiatrist cannot avoid communicating and at times imposing his own values upon his patients. The patient usually has considerable difficulty in finding the way in which he would wish to change his behavior, but as he talks to the psychiatrist his wants and needs become clearer. In the very process of defining his needs in the presence of a figure who is viewed as wise and authoritarian, the patient is profoundly influenced. He ends up wanting some of the things the psychiatrist thinks he should want. (Halleck, 1971, p. 19)

Bandura, himself, recognizes the inevitable intrusion of the therapist's values on the client's choice, but sees this as potentially less harmful than the insight therapist's value intrusion and imposition. He states:

> The change agent's role in the decision process should be primarily to explore alternative courses of action available, and their probable consequences on the basis of which clients can make informed choices. However, a change agent's value commitments will inevitably intrude to some degree on the goal selection process. These biases are not necessarily detrimental, provided clients and change agents subscribe to similar values and the change agent identifies his judgments as personal preferences rather than purported scien-

tific prescriptions. Much more serious from an ethical standpoint is the unilateral redefinition of goals by which psychotherapists often impose insight objectives (which mainly involve subtle belief conversions) upon desiring changes in their behavioral functioning. (Bandura, 1969, p. 112)

So the behavioral therapist counters the insight-oriented therapist's thrust, and points, rightly I believe, to the insight therapist's own value intrusion, an example of which can be seen in the following anecdote taken from Goldberg's work (1977), entitled *Therapeutic Partnership.* Goldberg writes, "When I asked an analyst acquaintance of mine whether she and her patients have some explicit agreement about what they are working on together in therapy, she gave me an incredulous look. This highly trained, intelligent, and kind friend tolerantly pointed out to me that 'neurotics don't know what they want! How do you expect them to work on goals in their analysis? Instead, I point out to them through my interventions what it is they are working toward' " (pp. 3–4). The therapist's attitude in the above example, besides patronizing, is blatantly paternalistic. Believing that the client suffers from illusions—the chief illusion being that "he thinks that what he thinks is his trouble really is his trouble" (London, 1964, p. 75)—is the epitome of paternalism and discounts the patient's *a priori* priority regarding his own feelings, thoughts, and goals.

It seems that both sides, actionist and insightist, intrude on the value choices that both in theory, and in print, usually reserve for the client. The actionist intrudes more directly, the insightist, more insidiously; but the outcome is similar. The client is being squeezed out of his responsibility "to give direction to his own existence":

> The client entering therapy suffers from an inability to address adequately his existential responsibility. It is a person's existential responsibility to give direction to his own existence. Without this direction a person suffers from a lack of experienced meaning in his existence. His suffering is exacerbated by the therapist's collusion in avoiding these concerns in their encounter together. . . . If the dialogue between the agents fails to elicit or unclearly elicits the objectives and goals for their coming together, such conduct begs the question of psychotherapy. It is imperative in my view that the reasons for being in a therapeutic encounter be clearly understood and agreed upon by both agents, not merely inferred by one or the other. (Goldberg, 1977, p. 3)

This existential position, trying to find an ethical footing between insightist and actionist end points, points to enlarging and sharing responsibility; partnership replaces paternalism as its watch word. Goldberg further writes, "For the client to become a more responsible and effective person, he needs to be given responsibility for collaborating in his own emotional growth. This endeavor requires a partnership between therapist and client" (p. 13).

Consent is that agreement marking the partnership. Consent is our power; we can give it, withhold it, or waive it.

> The common law protects one of our most fundamental values — the inviolability of the individual. As explained by Judge Cardozo, "[e]very human being of adult years and sound mind has a right to determine what shall be done with his own body. . . ." Under existing tort law, consent is the mechanism by which the client grants the therapist permission to invade his person for the purposes of treatment. The informed consent of the client is necessary to distinguish legally permissible medical intrusions from those which would subject a therapist to liability for an unauthorized "offensive touching" or the assault and battery of his client. Unless the therapist's action is privileged, "[i]t is the settled rule that therapy not authorized by the patient may amount to a tort — a common law battery — by the physician." (Friedman, 1975, p. 52. Copyright 1975 by the Arizona Board of Regents. Reprinted by permission.)

So it is our common-law right to consent, to say "yes" or "no," to accept treatment, or refuse it.

In addition to common-law protections, constitutional grounds for consent and our right to refuse enforced therapy may also be found. Samuel Warren and Louis Brandeis first enunciated a right "to be left alone." Brandeis, in his famous dissent in *Olmstead* v. *United States,* recognized man's spiritual nature, his feelings, and his intellect — and our right to protect ourself from unjustifiable intrusion, which he saw as a violation of the Fourth Amendment. In *Griswold* v. *Connecticut,* Justice Douglas spoke for a plurality of the court in articulating the notion of "zones of privacy," which are protected by the Ninth Amendment. To quote Friedman (1975) who quotes Douglas, "Justice Douglas stated that the concept of liberty includes, 'the autonomous control over the development and expression of one's intellect, interests, tastes, and personality'" (p. 58). The rights of mental privacy and mental autonomy, "a person's power to generate thought, ideas and mental activities — his freedom of mentation" (p. 58), finds support in *Whitney* v. *California* and *Stanley* v. *Georgia.* Friedman (1975) quotes Justice Marshall on this point: "Our whole constitutional heritage rebels at the thought of giving government the power to control men's minds . . . whatever the power of the state to control public dissemination of ideas inimical to the public morality, it cannot constitutionally premise legislation on the desirability of controlling a person's private thoughts" (p. 59).

Yet this right, like many rights, is not absolute, but bounded. Children, for example, have greater restraints placed on their power of consent: so a third grader's expressed dislike of school and desire to take a day, week, or year off may have very little effect on his actual 9 to 3 routine. The "mentally incompetent," those a legal hearing declared so, have lost their legal power of attorney to sign documents and make contracts; as a result their consent or refusal becomes legally meaningless. Also the alleged "mental patient," whose contact with reality and ability to give consent are questioned, is having his right to refuse treatment threatened from "underneath," by questioning his judgment and intelligence "to know" and, hence, to make *competent* and *informed* consent.

If this right is not absolute, but bounded by chronological, emotional, and intellectual extremes, then the state may, under some conditions, impose treatment. As Friedman (1975) writes, "Of course, if the client is hallucinatory, profoundly retarded, or very young, it is difficult to honor the principle that the client, rather than the behavior modifier, should select the goals of therapy. Thus, ethical considerations regarding personal choice are raised." (pp. 48–49)

OVERRULING OR UNDERMINING CONSENT

Two subsections ago, a section was concluded with a quote from Perry London on the actionist's focus on symptoms as opposed to the insightist's focus on meaning. The last sentence of that quote was the following: "It is perhaps less presumptuous of the doctor, when all is said and done, to treat the symptom with some disdain for its role in the total life of the patient, than to think too far ahead of its consequences" (London, 1964, p. 121). It is now time to think ahead to the consequences of therapeutic action taken in lieu of consent.

Give a therapist (be he actionist, insightist, or existentialist) his druthers and he will choose a contractual relationship as the basis for his therapeutic interactions with his client. It is a simpler, cleaner model to follow. It is less wearing on conscience. And it is less slippery. When one is looking for an ethical footing, these are not insignificant considerations.

We do not always get our druthers, however. Complications do arise. For example, many therapists work for an agency, be it state hospital, university counseling center, elementary school, or county mental health clinic. In addition, we have entered a therapeutic age of "third-party payments": insurance companies and health care plans may pick up the tab for treatment rather than the traditional model in which the client pays. These complications create difficulties for the therapist; one such difficulty is deciding who is his client—the payer of the bills, the payer of his salary, or the nominal client? Choices do come up in reality that throw the therapist into an ethical quandry. For example, a token economy program on a closed ward of a state hospital that shapes up and reinforces correct eating habits, toileting, hygiene, the grounds being kept clean, and quiet time being observed may seem commendable, even innocuous; yet who is the chief beneficiary? It can be argued that the hospital staff or ward personnel benefit as much if not more than the patients. If the token economy program is a research project, with aspirations of a publication emerging, perhaps the researcher is the chief beneficiary. Holland (1974) makes this point in his article entitled, "Political Implications of Applying Behavioral Psychology":

> The use of behavior modification then relates directly to existing power relationships . . . whether the psychologist is concerned or not, the growing use of contingency management in our society most often is in the service of our present elite.
>
> The relationship between psychologist and the recipient of behavior modification is not the traditional one of professional to client. The person or group of persons whose behavior is being modified may be controlled for the benefit of yet some other person or group. (p. 415)

Bandura (1969) too, speaks of power, and "whether the power to influence others is utilized for the advantage of the controller or for the benefit of the controllee" (p. 82).

So ignoring the consequences (long range or immediate) of control, failing "to think too far ahead of its consequences," courts disaster. In the actionist's "shortsightedness"—his focus on immediate cause–effect contingencies—he ignores the broader "social philosophy or some hypothetical moral order" (London, 1964, p. 124), which none of us are free of or freed of considering, personally or professionally. The actionist cannot fairly charge his insight brethren with "incognizance" in the area of contingency management, while he himself exercises incognizance in the areas of social, moral, and political consequences. London states it this way: "Indeed, the fact that he is so courageous (or stupid) as to himself assume responsibility for his work, must make him more alert to the implications it has for the social order and his own, as well as his patient's role in it" (pp. 124–125).

Something else seems to be happening; and it is subtler and more dangerous in many ways. The very nature of consent, the notions we have of it, are undergoing change, and the consequences of this changing outlook, although still unclear and far from final, nonetheless give off ominous tones.

"Consent" itself seems to be under attack from two sides, although "attack" may seem harsh and hyperbolic. Yet the right of consent is being challenged: challenged via the concept of *privilege*—which gives the "knowing best" and "acting in the best interest" role to the parent, state, physician, or therapist under certain circumstances; and challenged via the notion and image of the *child,* legally called *incompetency* but also fused and confused with *mental illness,* which psychologically sees the alleged patient as too childlike to know or incapable of making such therapeutic decisions as setting goals. The former challenge says, "I *know* best;" the latter challenge says, "he does not *know,*" or "he does not know enough to *know.*" (Someone is usually claiming that they *know,* while the other, merely knows.) The two challenges are linked and alike, however, in that the "parent–child" dance is being reenacted. Let us go through the steps.

"The doctrine of privilege," to quote Friedman (1975), "may protect a therapist from what would otherwise be deemed a tort. When the doctrine applies," and now Friedman quotes from a case note, "it signifies that the defendant has asked to further an interest of such social importance that [the interest] is entitled to protection, even at the expense of damage to the plaintiff. He is allowed freedom of action because of his own interests, or those of the public require it, and social policy will best be served by permitting it." Friedman goes on to add, "For example, consent is not required under tort law if there is an emergency, action in this situation being considered privileged. Thus, to the extent that statutes or judicial decisions sanction intervention by the therapist in certain circumstances, liability will not be imposed." Friedman adds a footnote here, which is germane: "For example, privileges protecting therapists and institutional employees from liability might be recognized in situations where an inmate is physically restrained for his own protection or the protection of other inmates. They also might be recognized in situations where physical contact is necessary to care for an incompetent patient." (pp. 54–55)

What Friedman is alluding to is emergency treatment, the image of the physician ministering to an unconscious auto-accident victim who is unable to give meaningful consent comes to mind. For a psychotherapist, the image may be one of overruling by coercion violence on the part of a patient. These are situations in which immediate harm to self or others, or an extreme risk, may be avoided by paternalistic interference. But may it also be sanctioning *extreme paternalism?* If we recall an early section, subtitled "The Meaning of Paternalism, and its Ethical Defenses," we recognize the principle of *extreme paternalism* (Robinson, 1974) being invoked, which is "the belief that the public at large lacks the discipline, motivation, and talent necessary to protect its own interests, even to learn its own interests. Arguments for a philosopher-King, for a benign dictator, for the State as suprapublic all rest on this principle" (p. 234).

This justification for coercion, therapeutic control taken in the absence of consent, invokes not the principle of *harm,* but of *ignorance*—implying that the plaintiff (and his cries may indeed be plaintive) does now know his best interest (e.g., like refusing to take his medicine), or a wider range of freedom can be had (e.g., engaging in successful toileting practices leading to freedom from diapers and a restricted ward schedule), or far-reaching decisions (e.g., long-term gains of sterilization or psychosurgery) are best made by paternalistic interference. The crossing line between legal and extreme paternalism may be at hand. "Do we cross?"

There is still a third challenge to consent. This one is a direct challenge, for it sees in the concept "willing consent," an "illusory criterion" (Bandura, 1969, p. 82). This point comes home in the *Kaimowitz* case.[2] The Kaimowitz case centered around psychosurgery, an experimental procedure that involves the surgical destruction or removal of brain tissue with the "intent of altering behavior" (Brown, Wienckowski, & Bivens, 1973). Specifically, a research project sponsored by the Lafayette Clinic and the Department of Mental Health for the State of Michigan was filed "For the Study of Treatment of Uncontrollable Aggression." The researchers wished to compare the effects of surgery "on the amygdaloid portion of the limbic system of the brain with the effect of the drug cyproterone acetate on the male hormone flow. The comparison was intended to show which, if either, could be used in controlling aggression of males in an institutional setting, and to afford lasting permanent relief from such aggression (sic) to the patient."[3] The experimental subjects were to be 24 criminal sexual psychopaths. One such subject was Joe Doe, who

---

[2] *Kaimowitz* v. *Michigan Department of Mental Health,* 42 U. S. L.W. 2063, 2063–64.

[3] Cited from the opinion, *Kaimowitz* v. *Department of Mental Health for the State of Michigan,* Civil Action No. 73–19434–AW, p. 3.

had been a resident of Ionia State Hospital for more than 17 years, committed there after being charged with murder and rape. John Doe signed the lengthy consent form which is reproduced in the footnote[4] below; but relatively soon thereafter, "Doe's view on the operation began to change."[5] He read literature critical of psychosurgery, and subsequently withdrew his consent. This brings us to our present point—his consent and its withdrawal—and to the broader questions of whether John Doe can give "legally adequate consent."

The issues raised in the Kaimowitz case involve three factors that underlie "legally adequate consent": competence, knowledge, and voluntariness. Is the subject competent to give consent? Does he have sufficient knowledge to make informed consent? Is his consent voluntary? Let us look at these three questions.

---

[4] "Since conventional treatment efforts over a period of several years have not enabled me to control my outbursts of rage and anti-social behavior, I submit an application to be a subject in a research project which may offer me a form of effective therapy. This therapy is based upon the idea the episodes of anti-social rage and sexuality might be triggered by a disturbance in certain portions of my brain. I understand that in order to be certain that a significant brain disturbance exists, which might relate to my anti-social behavior, an initial operation will have to be performed. This procedure consists of placing fine wires into my brain, which will record the electrical activity from those structures which play a part in anger and sexuality. These electrical waves can then be studied to determine the presence of an abnormality.

"In addition electrical stimulation with weak currents passed through these wires will be done in order to find out if one or several points in the brain can trigger my episodes of violence or unlawful sexuality. In other words this stimulation may cause me to want to commit an aggressive or sexual act, but every effort will be made to have a sufficient number of people present to control me. If the brain disturbance is limited to a small area, I understand that the investigators will destroy this part of my brain with an electrical current. If the abnormality comes from a larger part of my brain, I agree that it should be surgically removed, if the doctors determine that it can be done so, without risk of side effects. Should the electrical activity from the parts of my brain into which the wires have been placed reveal that there is no significant abnormality, the wires will simply be withdrawn.

"I realize that any operation on the brain carries a number of risks which may be slight, but could be potentially serious. These risks include infection, bleeding, temporary or permanent weakness or paralysis of one or more of my legs or arms, difficulties with speech and thinking, as well as the ability to feel, touch, pain and temperature. Under extraordinary circumstances, it is also possible that I might not survive the operation.

"Fully aware of the risks detailed in the paragraphs above, I authorize the physicians of Lafayette Clinic and Providence Hospital to perform the procedure as outlined above."

[5] Taken from the post-trial brief of Amicus Curiae; American Orthopsychiatric Association, p. 12.

COMPETENCE

Regarding competence, the Amicus Curiae brief (Note 5) states: "In the context of a mental patient's right to give an informed consent to a medical procedure, *competence* should mean the *capacity* to understand *rationally* the nature of the procedure, its risks and other relevant information. This formulation is an analogue of the legal tests to determine whether a person is competent to stand trial or to maintain his property" (p. 57). Let us look at John Doe's competence. For 18 years he lived in a hospital environment where "all major and most minor decisions were made for him, and the decision-making processes were arbitrary and incomprehensible" (p. 60). Previously, we have examined the effects of institutionalization (e.g., "the institutionalization syndrome" and "the social-breakdown syndrome") that decreased autonomy and increased dependency. John Doe's history for the last 18 years did not allow him the opportunity to make major decisions. Now he is asked "to make a decision of overriding importance on his own." The amicus "asks the court to recognize that, with respect to this decision, legally competent mental patients have diminished capacity and are peculiarly vulnerable, as a result of their mental condition, the deprivations stemming from involuntary confinement, and the effects of the phenomenon of 'institutionalization' " (Note 5, p. 62).

This argument seems to cut two ways and may, in fact, undercut the very power of the patient to consent, which the amicus brief is trying to defend. It seems to me that the more one asserts "incompetence" on the part of involuntary, long-term patients (although the point does not have to refer exclusively to involuntary patients) to make competent consent, or competent withdrawal of consent, the greater is the argument for "privilege" strengthened. The temptation is to conclude, "Well, then, let a guardian give consent." But the amicus group argues against this option, pointing out that others may not be acting in the "best interest" of the patient, may be promoting their own interests, or may be in conflict of interest. This can be seen if we hypothesize, for a moment, what might happen if a parent or hospital superintendent were to act as guardian and give consent in a case like John Doe's. What if the parent was the one who originally sought the commitment? Does he not have his own interests (e.g., safety) to protect? And what if the hospital superintendent is backing the research project? Does he not have his own interest in securing consent? We are back to third-party therapy problems, as the Amicus Curiae brief recognizes:

Second, doctors who are administering experimental "therapies" to research subjects have a conflict of interest which means that they may not be able to act solely in the patient's interest. Although they will want the patient to improve, they will, inevitably, also wish to advance science through pursuit of their own research interests. Accordingly, they may, consciously or unconsciously, exert psychological pressure on the potential subject to induce him to undergo an experimental medical procedure or cut corners in administering procedures designed to secure a fully voluntary consent. Such pressure may be especially prevalent when, as is the case here, the doctors are trying to fit patients into a research design. . . . Moreover, the possibilities of improper pressure are heightened when, as here, the research institution has received funds especially appropriated by the legislature for the particular research project and when trained staff and costly equipment await experimental subjects. (Note 5, p. 70)

If one's competence to consent is debatable, then the consent itself — its meaningfulness and legality — is thrown into doubt; but more, it is likely to be thrown to another — the paternalistic state, therapist, or guardian.

KNOWING

When we turn to the question of *knowing,* Justice Cardozo's remarks, quoted in the Kaimowitz opinion (Note 3), seem very apropos: "We are free only if we know, and so in proportion to our knowledge. There is no freedom without choice, and there is no choice without knowledge — or none that is illusory." Applying this to John Doe and other such patients, we could argue that consent is meaningless if you do not know what you have consented to; and a battery action can be brought against a doctor for not adequately *informing* his patient: a doctor must give the patient all the relevant information necessary to make a knowing (free) choice. Yet we might ask in the case of John Doe and his mentally ill kin, "Can he *understand* the information?" The amicus brief states, "It is extremely difficult for an involuntarily confined patient to give a *knowing* consent to experimental psychosurgery" (p. 64).

We are in troubled waters again. If the argument is that the mentally ill person does not have the intelligence to comprehend the meaning of stereotaxic surgery, mind-brain interactions, EEG, and microelectrode literature, I would, in turn, ask, "Who does?" Does not the argument extend to so-called normals as well? Outside of a few neurologists, neurosurgeons, and neuropsychologists, most of us would consent to surgery on *faith* rather than knowledge. Does not this argument extend to any complicated surgical procedure, such as neurosurgery or heart surgery? Could a mental patient give knowing consent to relieve a strictly medical situation? Could a mental patient, or normal hospital patient, give knowing consent when the procedure is complex?

If the argument is more discriminative, that is, arguing that normals can comprehend "enough" to make a "reasonable" judgment but involuntary, long-term mental patients cannot, then the burden of proof rests on those claiming the mental patient cannot know. Is it insufficient capacity, that is, low IQ? The literature would not support that claim. The claim that institutionalization decreases "the intellect" sufficiently to impair knowing, an assertion difficult to test experimentally,[6] also is not supported by empirical findings.

This argument based on "knowing," like the prior argument based on competency, seems to me to be a poor defense of the patient's right to refuse or consent; it undermines the very competency of the patient's consent, or withdrawal of consent; thus it adds further support to the forces and argument of privilege, paternalism, and third-party decision making as an alternative to the patient's "now questioned" capacities. The court opinion in Kaimowitz (Note 3) rejected the argument "that a truly informed consent cannot be given for a regular surgical procedure by a patient, institutionalized or not" (p. 21).

VOLUNTARY

The third issue relating to a legally valid consent is whether the consent was given voluntarily or not. Much of our legal thinking on this matter comes from the Nuremberg trials, and the code that emerged. In simple language and imagery we all recognize that a "shot-gun" wedding is not a voluntary consent. The groom (or bride, depending on whom the gun is trained) is not freely saying, "I do." The court of reason and law would be quick to disallow such enforced consents. Yet coercion comes in many forms, subtle as well as direct. Here is a passage from the Amicus Curiae (Note 5) brief: "As noted, the third requisite of a valid consent is that it must be *voluntary*. This requirement means that the potential research subject should be able to decide freely

---

[6] For example, if we documented that John Doe's IQ was 105 when he entered the hospital and 93 when measured now, is the drop of 12 points reliable and valid enough to conclude that "sufficient impairment" has resulted or that a current IQ of 93 is "insufficient" to weigh such weighty matters?

whether he wishes to undergo the experimental procedure, without the intervention of any overt *or indirect* element of force, fraud, deceit, duress, over-reaching, or other ulterior form of constraint or coercion" (p. 59).

Involuntary patients, like prisoners, are under extra pressures, sometimes stated, other times implied, to consent in order to be released or have their confinement shortened or improved. This is still coercion. Patients may be consenting to please their doctors, or because they fear reprisals if they do not consent. Their position in "an inherently coercive institutional environment" does not afford them the opportunity and freedom to " 'bargain' as equals with the doctors and administration over whether they should undergo psychosurgery" (p. 71).

A passage from the court's opinion (Note 5) summarizes the subtle problems of "voluntary" consent, and the dilemma it creates.

> Counsel . . . argues that anyone who has ever been treated by a doctor for any relatively serious illness is likely to acknowledge that a competent doctor can get almost any patient to consent to almost anything. Counsel claims this is true because patients do not want to make decisions about complex medical matters and because there is the general problem of avoiding decision making in stress situations, characteristic of all human beings. (p. 120)

Perhaps this is what Bandura had in mind when he said that the concept of "willing consent" was an "illusory criterion" (1969, p. 82).

Now we add to the dilemma the aspect of involuntary hospitalization. The court opinion (Note 5) adds, "Everything defendant's counsel argues militates against the obtaining of informed consent from involuntarily detained mental patients" (p. 21).

If hospital, doctor, stress, and complexity of procedure are operating (and conspiring) to turn a "seemingly voluntary consent" into something less, then the value, if not the very possibility of "freely given consent," is thrown into doubt and question.

Now we return to Skinner, smiling no doubt, who in his best determinist voice and reflex, kicks the concept of consent right in the teeth, and tells us, "Of course there is no *voluntary* consent!" The *response* of consent or refusal itself is *determined* by still other factors—the twins of past reinforcement history and genetic endowment—and not by any autonomous man exercising free will. "Consent," what we have been considering as the prelude and necessary prerequisite for a therapeutic response, is itself considered a *response,* and as such, subject to *control.* Where formerly consent sanctioned control and set a chain of responses in motion, now we have a different story: consent is not the "first cause," but a response that has its own antecedents—and controls: it is control, in some form, that spawns consent. "Consent," which has held a "sacred" and "mystical" place in the therapeutic cosmology, has been demystified; the "sacred" has become "profane;" and now it is seen as no less than, but *no more than,* any other response.

It is enough to make autonomous man shudder.

THE THERAPEUTIC CONSEQUENCES

So what are the therapeutic consequences of overruling or undermining consent? What happens when treatment is initiated in lieu of consent? We might, as a way of illustration, look at what typically happens when an actionist sets up a token economy program on a closed ward of a hospital, or sets up a behavior modification schedule for one particular patient. Usually, if the therapist knows his literature and controls the relevant parameters (e.g., type of schedule, type of reinforcers, interval of delay between response and reinforcement), the targeted behaviors can be shaped up or brought under greater environmental (therapist) control in all—save for the rare, "willful" patient. There are "those," of course—the resisters. But they are few; and their motivations, however quaint, confused, and fathomable, need not trouble us (although they may give us inspiration and insights, too); for we have so many successful cases to report. The literature is full of articles and anthologies documenting the control of such a variety of human behaviors that the citings would fill pages. That is not the point, however. The Insightist would be quick to grant the actionist his results; he might even yawn, or scowl, or raise an eyebrow, or all of these; but he would probably remain unimpressed by the demonstrations of behavior change, and might quip, "When you totally control someone's environment, of course you can get them to jump through hoops, eat their porridge, and apply underarm deodorant. Circus trainers have been demonstrating operant principles through their protegees' actions for centuries. So what is new about 'ward management' and 'B-mod'? If you can get the bear to apply underarm deodorant, do long division, and not engage in violent behavior *after* you have released him from your circus to his native habitat, then I would be impressed."

The Achilles heel of the actionist has just met Paris' arrow and force, guided by Appollo's vectoral direction: this is my way of raising the problem of *generalizability*. The actionist has gotten good *control* of behavior when he has *controlled* the environment, but change the environment, as when you discharge a patient from closed ward to community, and the behavior seems "out of control." If the behavior was, in the hospital environment, only under the therapist's (controller's) control—but not under *self*-control—then generalization is very unlikely.

Curiously enough, we have arrived back to the issue of consent once again, only this time the route has changed. Actionist's, however much they deterministically decry consent and its "free will" implications, need it. They need the patient's consent if generalization of behavior change to a new environment is to occur. The actionist, in Perry London's language, may present his client with a detailed blueprint for change that promises him wider freedom, yet the patient's cooperation is often "indispensable" if the plan is to be executed successfully. "These plans are not necessarily imposed arbitrarily upon the patient, and some therapists find it useful, even indispensable, to enlist the active cooperation of the patient in planning the treatment" (London, 1964, p. 79). This is *consent*.

Something is changing in the behaviorist camp, in its perspective and its rhetoric. Second and third generation actionist types are widening their world view of "behavior," "control," and "therapy." For example, Thoresen and Mahoney(1974) in their book *Behavioral Self-Control* (where the inclusion of the word "self" itself is a big change in the scheme of things) write: "Likewise, the term 'behavior' is defined very broadly—thoughts, feelings, and images are just as 'behavioral' as push-ups and conversation" (pp. 9–10). Those who have looked for so long at the "outer" are now coming to see the need for examining the "inner," and integrating the two. Again, Thoresen and Mahoney write:

> The paradigm of self-control presented here has minimized the long-standing traditional dichotomies such as internal versus external control and "self"-control versus environmental control. Such conceptions are anachronistic given what we now understand about human behavior. Clearly the exclusive inner-causation perspectives of many phenomenological orientations fail to account for the marked influence of external physical and social environments. Likewise, behavior conceptions that all but ignore the person's internal environment fall short by attributing all change to the external scene. The "in here" versus "out there" ways of thinking, lamented by Roszak (1969) and others, foster a conventional wisdom that has obstructed progress in solving the problems of self-control. (pp. 129–130)

110

Thoresen and Mahoney's conclusion is stated in their preface, "We have lacked and often denied the perspective that synthesizes the within and without, a view that sees self-control as a function of what goes on within the person, as well as things and events without. This deficit in turn has restricted development of a technology for teaching and learning the skills of self-control" (p. viii).

The skills and literature of self-control are growing. Also the relevance and relatedness of self-control to such concepts of freedom, choice, values, and therapy seem much more apparent now. We have primarily been relating self-control and choice to the decision involving the selection of therapeutic goals – those decisions requiring value judgments. Bandura (1969) had remarked that there were two basic decision systems, one regarding goals and values, and the other regarding specific procedures. Bandura thought that, "In the latter domain the agent of change must be the decision-maker, since the client is in no position to prescribe the learning contingencies necessary for the modification of his behavior," whereas in the former domain of goals and values, the client had the choice.

The self-control literature challenges Bandura's claim with evidence. When children are allowed choice, when they could select their own reinforcers and the contingencies for earning them, they performed better than when the identical reinforcers and contingencies were imposed by a teacher. Self-control and choice seem to be more rewarding than external regulation. Monkeys, cats, and rats[7] also demonstrate the motivational properties of choice. So here we see the therapeutic value of a client consenting, planning, and taking responsibility in carrying out his own treatment plan. It produces more demonstrable gains and more lasting changes than can be produced by externally imposed regulation.

To summarize the above points: the definition of "behavior" is widening to include the formerly "inner" events; and the importance of "control" is being refined to mine "self-control." Spinning those two threads together is Thoresen and Mahoney (1974), who quote from Goethe on their dedication page; it goes "Whatever liberates our spirit without giving us self-control is disastrous." We might add that the changing of responses, the discharging of feeling, or the flashes of insight will mean therapeutically little if self-control does not also occur. We see, then, that "therapy" becomes that process (conducted on inner and

---

[7] See studies cited by Thoresen and Mahoney (1974), p. 3.

outer levels by both therapist and client) of bringing about self-control on all levels.

Thoresen and Mahoney say, "The cardinal feature of self-control is that it is the person himself who is the agent of his own behavior change" (p. 11). Giving consent is the first act of self-control the agent makes, and the first step of the process of therapy. Consent lives! And it must, for therapy's sake, and more, for self-control's fate and meaning. Consent and self-control are wedded in common bond and source. For action in the name of therapy to be so in fact as well as in name, it cannot wrest control and consent from the client. We have learned from history and afresh through the problem of generalizability that if *you* take control, you are only going to have to give it back in the end. One has to heal the parent–child, reason–madness nexus, not widen it.

THE AFTERMATH AND IRONY—THERAPY
SEEN AS PUNISHMENT

When consent has been overruled, or when treatment has been involuntary, negligent, absent, or harsh, the courts have been asked with growing frequency to look into this therapeutic looking glass called "treatment" and see into its essence and truth: on some occasions, the courts have seen punishment. Increasingly, courts have used the expression "cruel and unusual punishment" in describing what defendants have called "treatment" or "therapy." Such treatments as "milieu," indefinite and involuntary hospitalization, electroconvulsive therapy (ECT), aversive conditioning, "time-out," isolation, seclusion rooms, contingency management, and psychosurgery have been challenged as being punishment rather than treatment.

Friedman (1975) cautions us, however, lest we think that the courts are rushing in to scrutinize questionable practices: he tells us of the court's historical reluctance "to employ the Eighth Amendment in the absence of particularly objectionable conditions. . . . Prior decisions have restricted the cruel and unusual punishment ban to those conditions which are 'barbarous' and 'shocking to the conscience,' and to physical and mental abuse or corporal punishment of such base, inhumane, and barbaric proportions so as to shock and offend a court's sensibilities" (p. 62). This limited and extreme view of *cruel and unusual* "may limit its applicability to many behavioral procedures."

On the other hand, Friedman notes a changing judicial view, one expressed by Justice Douglas in a dissent, that, if followed by the majority of the Supreme Court, would lead it to *greater* inspection of "therapeutically questionable treatments." Douglas said[8] "The delineation of just what conditions constitute cruel and unusual punishment is not well defined. But we know . . . that the concept is not rigid but progressive; that it acquires meaning as the public becomes enlightened."

One such case that illustrates the court's recent entree into "therapeutic territory and meaning" is *Knecht* v. *Gillman*[9]. The Eighth Circuit Court of Appeals "indicated that the Eighth Amendment also may protect mental patients from certain forms of enforced 'treatments' which have been imposed over their objection and which are really punishments in disguise. In this regard, the Eighth Amendment might be more accurately viewed not as an independent basis for a right to refuse treatment, but rather as a foundation for a collateral right to refuse hazardous or intrusive procedures which are only ostensibly treatment. This is the determinative issue in any Eighth Amendment challenge since the proscription applies only to punishment and would not provide a basis for challenging bona fide treatment, however painful it might be."

Friedman (1975) then goes on to describe the issues and findings in Knecht:

In *Knecht,* two residents of the Iowa Security Medical Facility (ISMF) sought to enjoin the use of apomorphine, a morphine base, vomiting-inducing drug, on nonconsenting residents. At ISMF, apomorphine was used as part of an aversive conditioning program for patients with behavioral problems. Under the ISMF program, "the drug could be injected for such pieces of behavior as not getting up, for giving cigarettes against orders, for talking, for swearing, or for lying." The patients at the facility who might be "treated" under this program included residents from any institution under the jurisdiction of the state department of social services, persons found to be mentally imcompetent to stand trial, referrals by the court for psychological diagnosis or as part of the pretrial or presentence procedure, and mentally ill prisoners.

The *Knecht* court found administration of apomorphine, in the absence of informed consent, to be cruel and unusual punishment. The court refused to accept ISMF's assertions that providing apomorphine as part of a "treatment" program exempted it from Eighth Amendment consideration, noting that "the mere characterization of an act as 'treatment' does not insulate it from Eighth Amendment scrutiny." The court then concluded that:

Whether it is called "aversive stimuli" or punishment, the act

---

[8] *McLamore* v. *South Carolina,* 409 U. S. 934, 934 (1972).

[9] 488 F. 28 1136 (8th Cir. 1973).

of forcing someone to vomit for a 15-minute period for committing some minor breach of the rules can only be regarded as cruel and unusual unless the treatment is being administered to a patient who knowingly and intelligently has consented to it. To hold otherwise would be to ignore what each of us has learned from sad experience — that vomiting (especially in the presence of others) is a painful and debilitating experience. The use of this unproven drug for this purpose on an involuntary basis, is, in our opinion, cruel and unusual punishment prohibited by the eighth amendment. (pp. 63–64)

Patients being forced to vomit was more than the Eighth Circuit Court could stomach. The practice, and the painful, personal memories struck the court's sensibilities. The court was willing in the *Knecht* case, "to look behind the mask of therapy and recognize when an objectional practice is punishment" (Friedman, 1975, p. 64).

Beyond the *Knecht* decision, *Wyatt,* v. *Stickney*[10] extends the court's scrutiny of enforced therapy into the very heart of behavior modification and token economy programs: typically, in such a therapy program, the patient is deprived of certain items or activities of value that are then given, contingent (following) on performing the desired responses. But the *Wyatt* court has drawn a distinction between absolute rights and contingent rights; under the court's decision patients are guaranteed, as absolute rights, a "comfortable bed, privacy, nutritionally adequate meals, the right to have visitors, to attend religious services, to wear their own clothes, to exercise regularly, to be out of doors regularly, and to interact with members of the opposite sex. As one commentator has noted: 'The crux of the problem, from the viewpoint of behavior modification, is that the items and activities that are emerging as absolute rights are the very same items and activities that the behavioral psychologists would employ as reinforcers — that is, as 'contingent rights'. . . . Thus, the usual target behaviors for token economies would be disallowed and the usual reinforcers will be legally unavailable" (Friedman, 1975, p. 75). The behavior modifier cay stay in business in at least two ways: he can switch to nonbasic reinforcers; that is, instead of denying a patient food until he makes the desired response, the inmate might be offered a choice of hard-boiled, soft-boiled, or scrambled eggs, for example, and then the most desired choice, but not the others, is made contingent upon the correct response (Goldfried & Davison, 1976); or, as another alternative, the behavior modifier can seek consent or a waiver of consent. The latter alternative, however, brings us back to familiar problems: "Who decides and

signs the consent or waiver form?" "The patient?" "The therapist?" "The hospital superintendent?" "Or community sentiment?" "Is the patient's consent or waiver valid?" Is it knowing,
voluntary, and competent?" For now, it is enough to restate the
questions.

What the court's action in *Wyatt* has done, taken together
with *Knecht, Kaimowitz,* and *Donaldson* (i.e., regarding "milieu
therapy" as a euphemism and a mask for no treatment), is afford
the patient greater guarantees to rights, proper treatment, and
powers to refuse treatment. Moreover the courts are showing
greater willingness to harness the controllers and scrutinize their
practices, in order to distill therapy from punishment.

If we asked the proverbial layman to define "therapy" and
"punishment," my bet is that he might have trouble putting his
thoughts into words, using technical terms properly, or giving
shading and nuance—but not with the basic meaning; thus he
might say that the terms are opposites—one helps and the other
injures, or one is undertaken in the name of rehabilitation, and
the other in the name of retribution. If the layman could be so
clear in his mind, why is the distinction so cloudy in ours? "So
cloudy," that Justice has been asked by litigators on behalf of
their clients to remove her blindfold and look into the haze, maze,
irony, and poignancy of "therapy–punishment." We who seek to
practice but not breach, ask, "How is it, that in the name of
benevolence, we seem to mix opposites—therapy and punishment
—to a point where the courts need all their alchemical powers to
separate sacred from profane?"

Here we have that irony again: a confusion of therapy with
punishment. More accurately, a confusion of therapy in the absence of consent (i.e., noncontractual therapy) with punishment.

Friedman (1975) speaks of the difficulty of separating therapy and punishment:

> While therapy and punishment properly defined may overlap to
> some extent, each is a distinct concept. Some genuine behavioral
> procedures may employ punishment to help a client extinguish
> certain behaviors, and many therapies may involve a great deal of
> physical or psychological pain, for example, "rolfing" or psychoan-
> alysis, respectively.
>
> The theoretical issue here is whether a finding of an Eighth
> Amendment violation can be based simply on the objective *impact*
> of a particular procedure or whether there also must be some find-
> ing of an *intent* to punish. (p. 63)

---

[10] 344 F. Supp. 373 and 387 (M.D. Ala. 1972), *aff'd subnom., Wyatt* v. *Aderholt,*
503 F. 2d 1305 (5th Cir. 1974).

We have, however, seen healers claiming that their *intent* is benevolent, albeit paternalistic, while the courts have disagreed. *Knecht* (Note 9) is the prime example. The court stated that "the mere characterization of an act as 'treatment' does not insulate it from Eighth Amendment scrutiny."

Wittgenstein would call this "language games."

Then there is Szasz (1970) and others, who are ready to rip the mask off other healers and their so-called "benevolent practices": "Oppression and degradation are unpleasant to behold and are, therefore, frequently disguised or concealed. One method for doing so . . . is to conceal the social realities behind the fictional facade of what we call, after Wittgenstein, 'language games' " (p. 133).

For us not to play "language games," therapists of all persuasions and shadings of actionist, insightist, existentialist, and what have you need agree on what therapy is: we who practice it ought to have a common ground. I suggest that, if "self-control" comes close to expressing the common ground, then certain actions suggest themselves, and certain implications follow regarding controls, values, and consent. The ethical thread can be heard and seen, in a metaphorical and literal way. It runs quite close and parallel to the therapeutic thread, and when that is recognized and coordinated, balance and harmony result in the change agent and client. If the common ground were held, *The Case for Controls* v. *The Right to Ruse Treatment* could be settled out of court, in our minds and hearts.

5

THE OPENING STATEMENT

In the famous contract scene from *A Night at the Opera,* Chico
Marx glares suspiciously at Groucho, points to some printed
words on the bottom of a now torn contract, and says, "What'sa
that?" Groucho, playing Otis B. Driftwood, says, "It's nothing. . . .
Just the sanity clause." Chico, who is nobody's fool, says, "You
can no foola me. . . . There is no sanity clause." When it comes to
sanity clauses, Chico and Groucho may both be right, or wrong, or
just plain confused. But then again, nobody else seems to be doing
any better.

When it comes to sanity and insanity clauses or defenses,
confusion still reigns. Historically, law makers have wrestled
with the confusing issue of insanity and the many questions surrounding it. How do you define insanity? And who defines it? Is an
insane person who commits a criminal act guilty in the *moral*
sense? Does he have an evil mind (*mens rea*)? Does he have free
will? Is he responsible? Should he be punished? Acquitted?
Treated? Increasingly in the last 200 years, philosophers, social
scientists, and mental health professionals have added their
voices, judgments, and presence to this evolving courtroom
drama, yet the results leave us no more clear than the Marx
Brothers did, and with much less humor. Life seems to be mirroring Art, in Marxian style; only nobody is laughing, save possibly
Groucho and Chico.

When psychologists and psychiatrists have entered the courtroom to tell *us*, the "ladies and gentlemen of the jury," whether

Insanity: Its Defenses, Defenders, and Detractors

the defendant is sane or insane, normal or abnormal, we often witness scenes that make us yearn for the "clarity" of the Marx Brothers. I have written about it this way (Finkel, 1976): "But the audience is catching on; it has witnessed too many cases in which both the defendant and the prosecution call 'experts' (all with impeccable credentials) in the mental health profession, who attest—with equal certainty and eloquence—that the accused is both perfectly normal and abnormal. As a result the profession is in danger of being convicted for lunacy" (p. 104). While the Marx Brothers do Dadist art and elevate comedy, the mental health profession does kitsch.

A recent article in the popular press (Newsweek, May 8, 1978) bearing the title, "Insanity on Trial," focused on the insanity defense, the growing public skepticism bordering on outrage regarding its use, and the debate over proposed remedies. From the "wild beast" test to the Durham decision, from M'Naghten to the American Law Institute's Model Penal Code, the legal definitions of insanity have *changed* over time; the 95th Congress of the United States had before it bills (S. 1437 and H.R. 2311) to codify and amend the Federal Criminal Code once again, and both bills have chapters dealing with "culpable states of mind" and "proof of state of mind" revisions; and yet, even as the definition of insanity stands on the verge of undergoing still further change, the public, political, and professional sectors wonder if we are any closer to the truth of the matter, or if we have *advanced* any from the beginning "wild beast."

We will, in this section, examine various insanity defenses

117

and their rationales, pointing out their respective strengths, weaknesses, errors, and ambiguities. This project could be a book in itself; it probably should be. This admission and forewarning alerts the reader that the topic will neither be covered fully, nor to the greatest depth possible. I have chosen to delimit some areas while highlighting others: the historical review of past insanity tests will be briefer than some readers may wish and focused more on *psychological* implications than legal. To be specific, the various insanity tests will be examined to show (a) their psychological understanding of man, and (b) their implications for the role of the mental health professional in this determination and drama. Hopefully this narrow focusing will allow greater resolution regarding our main topic — therapeutic ethics — while developing still further the themes of earlier sections.

THE WILD BEAST TEST

Since Roman law, men have held their peers responsible for their conduct; however, our judgement of our fellow men has been tempered by both mercy and reason: we continue to recognize "extenuating," "mitigating," and "exculpating" circumstances. For example, a man is exculpated for an offense if that offense results from self-defense. Besides self-defense, offenses that result from accident (where negligence is not a factor) have been similarly excused. A third example, one that is most pertinent here, is that men were not to be held accountable for offenses if the offense did not result from *free will*. This precedent for holding a man blameless if his action was not a willed action has been reestablishing itself in formulations of codes of conduct since Roman times.

In the eighteenth century, common law wrestled with the problem of codifying the diminishing responsibility applied to those whose actions seemed somehow not to be willed, particularly the actions of the insane. The first formulation relating criminality, responsibility, and insanity was the "wild beast" test. This test, formulated by Judge Tracy in *Rex* v. *Arnold*[1] in 1723, followed the line of reasoning of Lord Coke that relieved a man of criminal responsibility if he "doth not know what he is doing, no more than . . . a wild beast."

The test has as its virtue *simplicity*. It is easy for men of normal perception to tell a wild beast from a man. It was easy, for

---

[1] *Rex* v. *Arnold,* 16 How. St. Tr. 684, 764 (1723).

example, for the citizens of Paris in 1799 to agree that the wild boy (later to be known as "The Wild Boy of Aveyron") found in the woods by one Citizen Bonaterre (Itard, 1962) was a wild beast.[2] "What they did see was a degraded being, human only in shape; a dirty, scared, inarticulate creature who trotted and grunted like the beasts of the fields, ate with apparent pleasure the most filthy refuse, was apparently incapable of attention or even of elementary perceptions such as heat or cold, and spent his time apathetically rocking himself backwards and forwards like the animals at the zoo. A "man–animal," whose only concern was to eat, sleep, and escape the unwelcome attentions of sightseers" (pp. vi–vii).

Let us pretend, for a brief interlude, that one of the sightseers is none other than Voltaire, who happens to be carrying a copy of his latest book, and a loaf of fresh French bread. Let us further pretend that Voltaire passes close to the cage, too close, and the French bread is grabbed by the man–animal. Voltaire dives in to save his honor and bread, and a scuffle ensues. Voltaire is hit over the head with his book, his head and honor wounded, and the bread is gone. Voltaire brings charges of robbery, assault, battery, bad taste, and unfair literary criticism against the man–animal. The man–animal, through his court-appointed attorney, employs the insanity defense, claiming, in Judge Tracy's words, that "(my client) doth not know what he is doing, no more than . . . a wild beast." The Parisian jury would have no trouble deciding the case: "Not guilty, by reason of insanity."

The "wild beast" test's virtue, its simplicity, is also its disadvantage: it does not account for complex situations and tough discriminations. To decide that feral man (*Homo ferus*) is a wild beast and, hence, not responsible is easy, but not very applicable: there were only ten instances of Homo ferus reported from 1544 to 1731 (Itard, 1962). Yet the populace has realized that not every beast looks like a beast, and that there are "perfectly normal-looking" Dr. Jekylls hiding perfectly beastly thoughts within. The "wild beast" test gives us little help in discovering the wolf in sheep's clothing. The jury, also, who could not *see* into the man's interior, was often confused by the wide discrepancy between the defendant's court "appearance" and his alleged "actions." In their confusion, lay jurists were inclined to turn to "experts," — mental health professionals, psychiatrists, psychologists, seers, and divi-

---

[2] As an aside, Pinel, the famous physician of Bicetre and founder of moral treatment, disagreed with the masses as well as Itard, and thought the boy not to be a wild beast but an incurable idiot. So maybe it is not so easy for professionals to agree, even though the "common" judgment is in accord.

ners—the discipline whose history and press releases claimed insight into the "dark interior." The professional's intrusion into the courtroom was a century or two away, but the winds were already beginning to blow.

M'NAGHTEN

Many questions remained unanswered from the "wild beast" test. For instance, how do you determine how the defender's *knowledge* of the act compares to that of a wild beast? Do you ask him? And what if he declines to answer, as a wild beast might? If he is mute, inarticulate, or wild in responding, or if you suspect that he is faking, what then? Do you ask a professional to decipher? Does the authority in an insanity decision then shift from the jury to the professional? We will see these same questions arising in M'Naghten[3], and in our modern laws.

The "wild beast" test did undergo some modification. In 1760 (Leifer, 1964), the terms "right and wrong" were substituted for the original "good and evil." So the question turns on whether the alleged wild beast knows ethics and law, not morals. Although this shift focused the "knowing" on ethical rightness and legal correctness rather than on moral understanding and obedience, *know* the defendant must.

Another modification of the "wild beast" test resulted from the James Hatfield case, which occurred in 1800. It seems that Hatfield viewed himself as the new savior of mankind, who, like Jesus Christ, needed to become a sacrifice to attain his end; these were his "thoughts." To bring his aim about, he took aim at George III—but missed—wounding, instead, one of the King's attendants. Hatfield was defended most ably by Thomas Erskine, later to become the great Lord Erskine, who made a persuasive case for abandoning the "wild beast" test. Erskine claimed that Hatfield's "thoughts" suggested the "presence of a delusion," which acted as an "irresistible motive." Furthermore, Erskine presented evidence that Hatfield had suffered gunshot wounds to the head as a soldier in the service of the King. Putting these facts together and putting Erskine's defense in modern psychiatric language, it seems that Erskine was arguing that Hatfield's delusions resulted from an organic brain syndrome; thus, a bodily defect caused the delusion, which caused the defect of reason, which led to an irresistable motive, and to an uncontrollable act.

---

[3] Daniel M'Naghten's Case, 10 Cl. & Fin. 200, 8 Eng. Rep. 718, 1843.

Hatfield was acquitted, and the "wild beast" test seriously wounded.

The "wild beast" test, despite its problems and wounds, lasted for 120 years; then, in 1843, Daniel M'Naghten fired the shot that killed the "wild beast"; literally, he killed Edward Drummond, private secretary to the Prime Minister of England, Sir Robert Peel. The case becomes "interesting" rather than "just another routine London murder," because it was alleged "that Daniel M'Naghten 'was labouring under the insane delusion' of being hounded by enemies, among them Peel" (Szasz, 1970, p. 98). So it seems M'Naghten shot the wrong man, although there was some contention about that. Furthermore it was alleged that he thought he killed the right man, Peel. In short, M'Naghten was apparently suffering from a delusion that modern-day psychiatry might label paranoia.[4] According to Szasz, "Lord Chief Justice Tindal was so impressed by this evidence that he practically directed a verdict for acquittal. The jury found M'Naghten not guilty, on the ground of insanity" (p. 98).

The verdict incensed Queen Victoria. The politics and climate surrounding both M'Naghten and the Queen involved the Anti-Corn Law League plots, and a series of assassination attempts on the Queen's ministers, members of the English royal house, and once on Queen Victoria herself (*United States* v. *Currens*,[5] 1961, p. 763). The thought that such a "criminal" as M'Naghten might escape punishment on insanity grounds enraged the Queen. To quote again from Currens, "Public indignation, led by the Queen, ran so high that the Judges of England were called before the House of Lords to explain their conduct. A series of questions were propounded to them. Their answers, really an advisory opinion which were delivered by Lord Chief Justice Tindal for all fifteen Judges, save Mr. Justice Maule, constitute what are now known as the M'Naghten Rules" (p. 763).

The answers the Judges gave reduce to the following two rules, according to *Currens* (Note 5):

(1) "To establish a defense on the ground of insanity it must be clearly proved that, at the time of committing the act, the party accused was laboring under such a defect of reason, from disease of the mind, as not to know the nature and quality of the act he was doing, or if he did know it, that he did not know he was doing what was wrong." This rule was amplified with the comment that the knowledge of right and wrong refers to "the very act charged"

---

[4] *Hatfield*, 27 State Trials (1800); also cited in *Currens* (Note 5).

[5] *United States* v. *Currens*, 290 F.2d 751 (1961).

rather than to "knowledge" in the abstract. (2) "Where a person labors under partial delusions only and is not in other respects insane," and commits an offense in consequence thereof, "he must be considered in the same situation as to responsibility as if the facts with respect to which the delusion exists were real." (p. 764)

Those were the rules. It should be kept in mind that the justices were not actually formulating something brand new; in fact, the wording of the M'Naghten Rules can be found in the ancient book, *Eirenarcha,* which espoused the "right-wrong" doctrine more than 375 years earlier (Currens, Note 5). However, unlike *Eirenarcha,* the M'Naghten Rules took. As Currens noted, "These Rules have fastened themselves on the law of England and on the law of almost all of the States[6] and on all of the federal courts save one."[7]

Use of the M'Naghten Rules brought certain advantages over the "wild beast." Although the "wild beast" was a "simple" test, requiring a discrimination between normal man and a man who, for whatever reason, acts and knows no better than a wild beast, it did not speak to "insanity *within* domestic and familial boundaries." In answer to the question, "How much insanity must there be for someone to be judged legally insane?," the "wild beast" test admits and defines only extreme cases. As the community of men came to recognize insanity "closer to home," so to speak, they needed a new definition that would fit these less extreme, but more problematic, cases. M'Naghten provided the *specifics* that the simplistic "wild beast" test had lacked.

Some of the specifics can be seen in the phrases it uses: "defect of reason," "disease of mind," "nature and quality of the act," "did not know," and "did not know he was doing what was wrong." If Daniel M'Naghten had been tried under the "wild beast" criteria, his lawyer would have to make the case that whatever aspect differentiates man from lower beasts (e.g., call it a *ration,* the human essence, or soul, if you like), it is substantially diminished or absent in this particular case. Under the M'Naghten rules the key quality in question is his *reason;* of all of man's qualities, and we could mention will, emotions, imagination, and so forth, it is his *reason* and his *reason* only that is essential in the insanity determination; so one implication of M'Naghten regarding the early nineteenth century's psychological understanding of man is that *reason* has become the paramount defining aspect of psychological man.

---

[6] Except New Hampshire.

[7] The Court of Appeals for the District of Columbia Circuit.

The M'Naghten Rules also speak of "disease of mind," the cause of reason's defect; with these words, the province of psychiatry and psychology come to have direct bearing on the matter at hand, or, at least, its underlying condition, whereas in the "wild beast" test, professional opinion and disease of mind were not necessary.

With phrases like "to know the nature and quality of the act he was doing," M'Naghten again specified what the "wild beast" left vague. "To know" is both a complex verb and act, since varying degrees of "knowing" are possible. So what does it mean for the defendant to "know" what he is doing? Does it mean as little as having sensory awareness of his movements during the crime? Must it only be shown that M'Naghten was aware that he held a gun instead of a guava melon, and that he knew it was the former that he squeezed? Or is more required under the verb "to know"? Must M'Naghten also recognize that his act was infringing on another? Even causing pain and death? Must he further recognize that that is a criminal act? That it is legally impermissible? Or must he further recognize that it is morally wrong? Must M'Naghten *know* the criminality and immorality of his act? These questions serve to show the degrees of knowing that are possible, and anticipate the problems that post-M'Naghten juries would have in making such a determination. In comparison to the "wild beast" test, however, *knowing* has been defined more precisely ("nature and quality of the act"), at least in words. Whether we can *infer* the defendant's *degree of knowing* is quite another matter.

Problems with M'Naghten were many. Some were immediate. For one, and this was a major one, M'Naghten held to a psychological view of man that was being questioned *at that time;* men of eminence, like Dr. Isaac Ray for example, the American psychiatrist whose views led, in part, to New Hampshire's refusal to adopt the M'Naghten Rules, questioned the correctness of the M'Naghten view of insanity. In fact, as a footnote from Currens (Notes, p. 770) reveals, "When Cockburn defended Daniel M'Naghten, he frequently referred to a treatise on criminal insanity written by the eminent American psychiatrist, Isaac Ray."

What resulted from the M'Naghten Rule's overweighing of the intellect was that psychiatric testimony became correspondingly overweighted. For who else *seemed* expert at assessing both "disease of mind" and "intellectual impairment"? Yet these assumptions, one of Reason's hegemony, and the second that psychiatric testimony is expert testimony, are both questionable. Leifer (1964) is one who challenges these assumptions:

The McNaghten Rule *asserts* that responsibility is a function of the intellect: Reason is aligned with responsibility, and defect of reason is aligned with nonresponsibility. The key to the determination hinges on an evaluation of the "intellect" of the accused, specifically on whether he *knows* the nature and quality of his act and whether he *knows* that what he was doing was wrong. The job of the psychiatric expert witness is to aid the court in making this determination. For the psychiatrist to be considered an expert, he must have special skills or special knowledge which enable him to determine whether or not "Mr. Jones knows X," for which the "right and wrong" test offers specific instances.

Much like the medical pathologist or internist, the psychiatrist is considered to be a scientific expert, whose special province is the mind and the personality. Thus, it is thought that the psychiatrist has special skills and tools which enable him to penetrate the mind much as the toxicologist has special skills and tools for examining the blood. . . . However, there are differences between the psychiatrist and the toxicologist.

First, the determination that "Mr. Jones knows X" is an ordinary determination which most people make every day of their lives. Every day teachers determine whether their students know their work, employers determine whether their workers know their jobs, and mothers determine whether children know their manners. Such judgments do not require special skills. . . . Some special techniques might be required for eliciting the behavior on which a judgment is based, that is asking the proper questions, but interviewing is not a skill which the psychiatrist monopolizes. A skillful lawyer, detective, or personnel manager, among others, may be equally skillful in interviewing. . . .

Second, the judgment of whether or not "Mr. Jones knows X" is an ordinary one precisely because it is based on a knowledge of language usage, which most people possess. On the other hand, the judgment about the blood level of arsenic is based on the understanding of the specialized subjects of chemistry and physiology. (pp.825–826)

If Leifer's point is accurate, then we do not need a psychiatrist, psychologist, or mental health "expert" to ask the question, because the question is asked in ordinary language, requiring neither specialized subjects nor monopolized interviewing skills. In fact, Leifer cites two opinions in a footnote (1964, p. 826), one of which says, "A simple way of finding out is to ask the offender whether he now thinks his act is right or wrong," while the other states, "It must be apparent that the only direct way one can determine whether the accused has 'knowledge' of right and wrong is to place the question to him." In both of these remarks, the "expert" is out of the picture. Yet history reveals that he moved steadily into the picture, to where he now stands to be the central·character and witness in this drama, if not being accused himself of improper practices. From Cockburn citing Isaac Ray at M'Naghten's defense (1843), a rising stream of "forensic psychiatrists" and other "experts" have come through the court. As Leifer (1964) states:

> The use of a "scientific expert" to aid in the determination of responsibility eases the burden of the court by giving the impression that the determination rests on a scientifically determined fact rather than on an ambiguous matter of semantics. It thus disguises and distracts us from the fact that the courts have to justify life and death decisions on the basis of arbitrary and ambiguous criteria and provides what appears to be a scientific justification for the court's decision. Psychiatrists have been all too eager to testify, and why not? They have everything to gain and nothing to lose by it. In exchange for helping the court out of its difficulty, the psychiatrist's own claim to scientific status is underwritten by the courts. (p. 827)

Leifer points to an unwholesome collusion that has existed between courts and professionals. In fairness, however, he also reports the professional criticism of M'Naghten and "expert" testimony:

> These difficulties have been recognized by psychiatrists who have criticized the M'Naghten Rule since its inception. In two recent polls, more than 85% of the psychiatrists questioned disapproved of this test. . . . Philip Roche (1958) states: "The tests of responsibility as expressed in the M'Naghten Rule . . . are untenable propositions within the discipline of scientific medical psychology". . . . Gregory Zilboorg (1949) goes further: "To force a psychiatrist to talk in terms of the ability to distinguish between right and wrong and of legal responsibility is — let us admit it openly and frankly — to force him to violate the Hippocratic oath, even to violate the oath he takes as a witness to tell the truth and nothing but the truth, to force him to perjure himself for the sake of justice." *The fact that psychiatrists have willingly testified and continue to testify in tests of responsibility in spite of these criticisms and hazards can be explained by the social advantages, in terms of money, prestige, and power, that accrue to psychiatrists and to the institution of psychiatry as a result of this activity.* (p. 827)

Pretty strong stuff; but the final word, an irony at that, goes to a quote from *Currens* (Note 5), which summarizes the psychiatrist, his testimony, and his "gain" in an apt style: "All in all the M'Naghten Rules do indeed, as has been asserted so often, put the testifying psychiatrist in a strait-jacket" (p. 767).

AN IRRESISTIBLE IMPULSE

Mr. Justice Frankfurter, in his testimony in 1953 before the Royal Commission on Capital Punishment (*Currens*, Note 5) minced no words, making it plain that he thought the M'Naghten Rules were a sham:

> The M'Naghten Rules were rules which the Judges, in response to questions by the House of Lords, formulated in the light of the then existing psychological knowledge. . . . I do not see why the rules of law should be arrested at the state of psychological knowledge of a time when they were formulated. . . . I am a great believer in being as candid as possible about my institutions. They are in large measure abandoned in practice, and therefore I think the M'Naghten Rules are in large measure shams. That is a strong word, but I think the M'Naghten Rules are very difficult for conscientious people and not difficult enough for people who say, "We'll just juggle them" . . . I dare to believe that we ought not to rest content with the difficulty of finding an improvement in the M'Naghten Rules (pp. 765–766)

Men have been looking for improvements on M'Naghten ever since Queen Victoria scowled and shook her head in disbelief. One corrective to M'Naghten was the addition of volitional test. This test absolves an offender who knew what he was doing, knew that what he was doing was wrong, but who was unable, because of his mental condition, to refrain from doing so. This is sometimes referred to as the "irresistible impulse" test; however, it is probably wiser to call it simply a "control test" ("self-control" might be even more apropos) or "volitional test," since "irresistible impulse" implies a certain suddenness of motivation, a state of passion, not required by the test. Historically, the seeds of the irresistible impulse test could be seen in Erskine's defense of Hatfield (Note 4), when he asserted that Hatfield's delusions created "motives irresistible."

On the level of psychology, *will* is added to *reason* as a condition for sane behavior. As psychological knowledge advanced, and *will* became an important aspect of man and focus of study, the law responded and followed step, moving to a rule more consistent with the knowledge of the new time. As it was put in *Smith* v. *United States*[8] in 1929:

> The modern doctrine is that the degree of insanity which will relieve the accused of the consequences of a criminal act must be such as to create in his mind an uncontrollable impulse to commit

---

[8] *Smith* v. *United States*, 1929, 59 App. D.C.

the offense charged. This impulse must be such as to override the reason and judgment and obliterate the sense of right and wrong to the extent that the accused is deprived of the power to choose between right and wrong. . . . The accepted rule in this day and age, with the great advancement in medical science as an enlightening influence on this subject, is that the accused must be capable, not only of distinguishing between right and wrong, but that he was not impelled to do the act by an irresistible impulse, which means before it will justify a verdict of acquittal that his reasoning powers were so far dethroned by his diseased mental condition as to deprive him of the will power to resist the insane impulse to perpetrate the deed, though knowing it to be wrong.

This addition of the "irresistible impulse test" to the M'Naghten test was favored by those who saw it as more humane than M'Naghten alone, since it spared from retributive punishment those who were powerless to do other than commit the crime: this preserved and put into practice a key concept — that nondeterrables should be exculpated. In addition, it was favored by those who were oriented toward *treatment* rather than *punishment* of offenders who get "out of control." If they were treated in mental hospitals rather than sent to prison, we could have *incapacitation,* the virtue of prison, along with treatment and the chance of *cure,* the promise of mental health through hospitalization.

The control test has been extensively criticized. One criticism says that the test may exculpate offenders whose lack of resistance to the criminal urge may well have been a simple *failure* to resist, and not a real *inability* to resist the urge. Undertones of "free will" versus "determinism" and "conscious" versus "unconscious" motivation can be heard in this argument. Was the offender's lack of resistance a result of disease such that he was *unable* to resist, and hence the crime was caused? Or was the offender able to override whatever environmental and genetic factors were existing at the time, but refused — that is, he set his will, and made the conscious choice not to resist? This indeterminacy regarding the nature of the offender's lack of resistance creates problems and loopholes for courts and deterministic psychiatrists. Yet it is just this "impracticable" distinction that juries are asked to make.

We do want juries to tell us whether the lack of resistance to the criminal act results from true incapacity or mere indisposition. Given a difficult, if not impossible, discrimination to make, juries and courts are apt to beg the question and seek "professional" assistance. Enter the "expert" witness, again. Although the job of deciding sanity or insanity rests with the jury in theory, in practice it is the psychiatrist's testimony that offers to solve the Sphinx's maddening riddle, while relieving the court and jury of its dilemma, and responsibility. In believing that the professional has the power, expertise, and vision to penetrate the impenetrable, or to "see" where men and women (the judge and jury) of normal perception cannot Justice truly blindfolds herself. That, perhaps, is another form of insanity. As for the oracle, the professional, expert witness who models in modern contexts and courtrooms Oedipus' eye-opening pronouncement of an earlier age — let him remember his ancestor's fate, and hindsight.

THE DURHAM DECISION

Much trouble was brewing with M'Naghten and the "irresistable impulse" addition: for one, they no longer fit the existing state of psychological knowledge of the current, "new time." Man was no longer being *seen* as part reason, part will, and so on, but as a whole. Another difficulty with M'Naghten, which chiefly plagued the psychological expert witness, was the phrase "at the time of committing the act"; expert witnesses were seldom on hand at the scene of the crime, so examination of the defendant would most likely be an after-the-fact matter. Whether the psychiatric evaluation was done hours, days, weeks, or months after the event, the expert would still have to make *an inference* back to that earlier time of committing the act. Even if there was an earlier psychiatric evaluation, earlier than the crime let us say (e.g. as a hypothetical example, let us imagine that one year prior to the act the defendant was examined and hospitalized in a psychiatric institute), we would still be making inferences regarding the time of the act. No, neither before-the-fact nor after-the-fact psychiatric evaluation can speak with *certainty* regarding "the time of the act."

The resulting Durham decision and rule address both of these objections — objections to the conception of psychological knowledge of man that underlies the earlier test and to the after-the-fact applicability inference problem — and attempt to create a rule that harmonizes knowledge and testimony. The result has been disharmony (Leifer, 1964; Szasz, 1970; *United States* v. *Currens*, Note 5). Here is the story in brief.

According to Judge Bazelon (*Durham* v. *United States*,[9] "Monte Durham was convicted of housebreaking by the District Court sitting without a jury. The only defense asserted at the

---

[9] *Durham* v. *United States*, 1954, 214 F. 2d 862.

trial was that Durham was of unsound mind at the time of the offense. We are now urged to reverse the conviction (1) because the trial court did not correctly apply existing rules governing the burden of proof on the defense of insanity, and (2) because existing tests of criminal responsibility are obsolete and should be superseded" (p. 864).

Monte Durham had a history of mental illness, which showed an "on-again off-again" pattern. In 1945, at age 17, he was discharged from the Navy following a psychiatric examination that said he suffered "from a profound personality disorder which renders him unfit for Naval service." In 1947, he pleaded guilty to violating the National Motor Theft Act and was placed on three-year probation. In the same year, he attempted suicide and was transferred to St. Elizabeth's Hospital. He was discharged after two months. In January of 1948 he was convicted of passing bad checks. "His conduct within the first few days in jail led to a lunacy inquiry in the Municipal Court where a jury found him to be of unsound mind. Upon commitment to St. Elizabeths, he was diagnosed as suffering from 'psychosis with psychopathic personality.' After 15 months of treatment, he was discharged in July 1949 as 'recovered' and was returned to jail to serve the balance of his sentence. In June 1950 he was conditionally released." Already we can see the on-again off-again nature of his disorder: sometimes he is "fit" and "recovered," and at other times "unfit" and "psychotic."

The pattern continued after he was released. A violation of parole, a warrant for his arrest, flight to the south and midwest, and passing bad checks followed. Upon his return, the parole board referred him to the district court "for a lunacy inquisition, wherein a jury again found him to be of unsound mind. He was readmitted to St. Elizabeth's in February 1951. This time the diagnosis was 'without mental disorder, psychopathic personality.' He was discharged for the third time in May 1951. The housebreaking which is the subject of the present appeal took place two months later, on July 13, 1951."

There is more. "According to his mother and the psychiatrist who examined him in September 1951, he suffered from hallucinations immediately after his May 1951 discharge from St. Elizabeths. Following the present indictment, in October 1951, he was adjudged of unsound mind . . . 'psychosis with psychopathic personality.' He was committed to St. Elizabeth's for the fourth time and given subshock insulin therapy. This commitment lasted 16 months . . . when he was released . . . 'mentally competent to stand trial" and . . . able to consult with counsel to properly assist in 'his own defense.' "

Monte Durham was convicted, as his defense of insanity was rejected. The rejection was pure M'Naghten — there was no evidence of unsound mind as of July 13, 1951 — the time of the act. We have psychiatric "evidence" before and after the fact, but not at the time of the act. Also the evidence from before is equivocal: sometimes he had his psychosis and sometimes not.

Here is verbatim question and answer from his trial; Mr. Ahern is defense counsel and Dr. Gilbert is the expert witness giving psychiatric testimony (*Durham,* Note 9):

(1) Q. (Mr. Ahern). As a result of those examinations did you reach a conclusion as to the sanity or insanity of the defendant? A. Yes, I did arrive at an opinion as to his mental condition.

Q. And what is that opinion? A. That he at that time was of unsound mind.

Q. Can you tell us what disorder he was suffering from, Doctor? A. The report of his case at the time, as of October 9, 1951, I used the diagnosis of undifferentiated psychosis, but according to the record the diagnosis at the time of commitment psychosis with psychopathic personality.

Q. At that time were you able to make a determination as to how long this condition had existed? A. According to the record I felt at the time that he had been in that attitude or mental disorder for a period of some few to several months.

(2) Q. (Mr. Ahern). Directing your attention specifically to July 13, 1951, will you give us your opinion as to the mental condition of the defendant at that time? A. From my previous testimony and previous opinion, to repeat, it was my opinion that he had been of unsound mind from sometime not long after a previous release from Saint Elizabeth's Hospital (i.e., May 14, 1951).

(3) Q. (Mr. Ahern). In any event, Doctor, is it your opinion that that period of insanity would have embraced the date July 13, 1951? A. Yes. My examination would antedate that; that is, the symptoms obtained, according to my examinations, included that — the symptoms of the mental disorder. (Note 9, pp. 866–867)

So the expert witness is making an *inference.* The court in the original case remained unimpressed. They said:

I don't think it has been established that the defendant was of unsound mind as of July 13, 1951, in the sense that he didn't know the difference between right and wrong or that even if he did, he was subject to an irresistible impulse by reason of the derangement of mind. . . . *There is no testimony concerning the mental state of the defendant as of July 13, 1951, and therefore the usual presumption of sanity governs.* (Note 9, pp. 865–866)

The court of appeals thought this was an error requiring reversal. Here is part of their reasoning regarding psychiatric testimony not being "at the time of the act." "The inability of the expert to give categorical assurance that Durham was unable to distinguish between right and wrong did not destroy the effect of his previous testimony that the period of Durham's 'insanity' embraced July 13, 1951. It is plain from our decision in Tatum that this previous testimony was adequate to prevent the presumption of sanity from becoming conclusive and to place the burden of proving sanity upon the Government" (Note 9, p. 868). So the court is willing to embrace the expert's "opinion" that the defendant's "insanity" embraced the date in question; this in the face of the defendant's history of "on-again off-again insanity"; now the expert "feels sure" that on the date in question, his "insanity" was "on again"; or, as the court quaintly terms it, this "expert" testimony counts as "some evidence."

"Some evidence" indeed. This "little bit" of evidence tips the larger scale and changes the burden of proof. Yet this very decision, one which later cites Isaac Ray's 1838 edition of *Medical Jurisprudence of Insanity* in a footnote (p. 870, 22), seems to overlook Ray's words. Ray said, "That the insane mind is not entirely deprived of this power of moral discernment, but in many subjects is perfectly rational, and displays the exercise of a sound and well-balanced mind is one of those facts now so well established, that to question it would only betray the height of ignorance and presumption." From Ray's remarks, we may infer "with equal certainty," it seems to me, that Durham may well have been possession of his power of moral discernment, that he may have been "rational enough" to break into a house — but was "unlucky enough" to get caught.

So although there is a hunch (I prefer "hunch" as opposed to "some evidence") that he might have been insane, there is also another hunch that he was sane. The Appeals Court, in going with the first hunch, makes the burden of proof heavier for the prosecution, while it simultaneously lightens the psychiatric proof of insanity that is necessary. A psychiatrist testifying under M'Naghten Rules must produce evidence regarding the defendant's mental state and responsibility at the time of the act; a psychiatrist testifying under Durham rules need only produce hunches embracing the time of the act. The "quality" of the evidence has indeed changed — it has diminished — as the court is aware of, in its diminutive language, "some evidence." It may be small, but it is no little matter.

Durham did more than upset the balance of proof; it went to the underlying model of Psychological Man embedded in M'Naghten plus the impulse addition, and found it to be a relic — no longer appropriate to the "new time." Here is a quote from Durham (Note 9):

The science of psychiatry now recognizes that a man is an integrated personality and that reason, which is only one element in that personality, is not the sole determinant of his conduct. The right-wrong test, which considers knowledge or reason alone, is therefore an inadequate guide to mental responsibility for criminal behavior. As Professor Sheldon Glueck of the Harvard Law School points out in discussing the right-wrong tests, which he calls the knowledge tests:

"It is evident that the knowledge tests unscientifically abstract out of the mental make-up but one phase or element of mental life, the cognitive, which, in this era of dynamic psychology, is beginning to be regarded as not the most important factor in conduct and its disorder. In brief, these tests proceed upon questionable assumptions of an outworn era in psychiatry." (p. 871)

The court in *Holloway* v. *United States*[10] (1945) said: "The modern science of psychology . . . does not conceive that there is a separate little man in the top of one's head called reason whose function it is to guide another unruly little man called instinct, emotion, or impulse in the way he should go." A third view, the Royal Commission Report,[11] said "The gravamen of the charge against the M'Naghten Rules is that they are not in harmony with modern medical science, which, as we have seen, is reluctant to divide the mind into separate compartments – the intellect, the emotions and the will – but looks at it as a whole and considers that insanity distorts and impairs the action of the mind as a whole." So here are three eminent opinions, all finding M'Naghten's "Psychology" to be dated. Separate aspects of the mind, personified in thought and concretized and localized in the brain, were out; what was in, was a holistic, dynamic view of man.

The Appeals Court followed an 1870 New Hampshire ruling,[12] and formulated a sentence that came to be known as the Durham rule: "It is simply that an accused is not criminally responsible if his unlawful act was the product of mental disease or mental defect" (pp. 1874–875). The court went on to formulate rough instructions to the jury, that went like this:

If you the jury believe beyond a reasonable doubt that the accused was not suffering from a diseased or defective mental condition at the time he committed the criminal act charged, you may find him guilty. If you believe he was suffering from a diseased or defective mental condition when he committed the act, but believe beyond a

---

[10] *Holloway* v. *United States,* 1945, 80 U.S. App. D.C. 3, 5, 148 F. 2d 665, 667, certiorari denied, 1948, 334 U.S. 852, 68.

[11] Royal Commission on Capital Punishment, 1949–1953, Report (Cmd. 8932) 79 (1953).

[12] *State* v. *Pike,* 1870, 49 N.H. 399.

reasonable doubt that the act was not the product of such mental abnormality, you may find him guilty. Unless you believe beyond a reasonable doubt either that he was not suffering from a diseased or defective mental condition, or that the act was not the product of such abnormality, you must find the accused not guilty by reason of insanity. Thus your task would not be completed upon finding, if you did find, that the accused suffered from a mental disease or defect. He would still be responsible for his unlawful act if there was no causal connection between such abnormality and the act. These questions must be determined by you from the facts which you find to be fairly deducible from the testimony and the evidence in this case. (Note 12)

Standing back from the rule and its instructions for a moment, we might better see its promise and pitfalls. On the promising side, Durham changes M'Naghten's Psychology to what fits the "new time": the legal definition of responsibility changes from a competent intellect to a well-integrated personality; but there is a pitfall here, if we are not careful. Leifer (1964) says, "By bringing the test for criminal responsibility up to date with psychiatric theory, it was assumed that the ascription of responsibility was made more scientific. In fact, however, ascriptions of any sort, although they may be based on a consideration of facts, are themselves neither facts nor scientific principles; rather, they are human actions similar to 'giving' or 'bestowing' and as such are neither true nor false, and, therefore, cannot be considered to be scientific" (p. 827). What has happened *in fact* is just what the justices writing the opinion in Durham hoped would not. To continue Leifer's point, "The primary effect of the Durham Decision is to make the psychiatrist more comfortable with his testimony; he may now speak with the widest latitude, in his own parlance, using his own theories" (p. 828).

The Durham court's (Note 9) last words were as follows:

Finally, in leaving the determination of the ultimate question of fact to the jury, we permit it to perform its traditional function which, as we said in Holloway, is to apply "our inherited ideas of moral responsibility to individuals prosecuted for crime. . . ." Juries will continue to make moral judgments, still operating under the fundamental precept that "our collective conscience does not allow punishment where it cannot impose blame." But in making such judgments, they will be guided by wider horizons of knowledge concerning mental life." (p. 876)

Leifer (1964) sees the juries being guided and *misguided* more and more by psychiatrists. Leifer's point is quoted below:

Psychiatrists frankly admit this advantage and promote it, although they define it as primarily for the advantage of the court, whom they feel can now legitimately receive all of the information the psychiatrist is capable of giving. The absurdity of this euphemism is that it is the rare jurist or juror who can understand what the psychiatrist has to tell him (Wiseman, 1961). This "technicalization" of psychiatric testimony has resulted in the paradox that although one of the purposes of the Durham Decision is to insure that the moral decision is made by the jury rather than the expert, the facts on which that decision is to be based are so technical that the jury must hear the psychiatrist's conclusion as to whether the act was a product of mental disease or not, which is equivalent to an opinion about responsibility. Far from making their own decision the jury can only agree or disagree with one of two psychiatrists, each of whom presents technical language which the jury cannot understand. Thus, it tends to be the psychiatrist, rather than the facts, that influences the jury; the effect is that the moral decision is placed more firmly in the hands of the psychiatrist, although more subtly. (p. 828)

WHAT KIND OF ILLNESS IS "MENTAL ILLNESS?"

From 1723 (the "wild beast") to 1954 (Durham), the psychiatrist has come to play the central, if not determining, role in the insanity drama; this fact is even more startling when we remember back to the "wild beast" beginnings and to the question of "knowing" — which required no special "expertise" to ask or decipher; now we have come from "knowing" through "defect of reason from disease of the mind" to "mental disease or mental defect," and the results have been a "technicalization" of language, a blurring of the distinction between "hunches" and "facts" and a confusion between correlational and causal relationships.

My goal here is to simplify things. Unfortunately, it has to get more complex before it gets simpler. The path takes us to the concept of mental illness, and the question, "What kind of illness is 'mental illness'?"

Within the mental health discipline, the term "mental illness" is used to describe two kinds of illnesses: (a) its minor usage is as a description of syndromes (i.e., groups of behaviors that occur together with some regularity) that correlate with organic, physical damage or destruction (e.g., the organic brain disorders, associated with intercranial damage, brain tumor, poison, nutritional deficiencies and the like, and the psychophysiological disorders, such as ulcer or collitus, for example) to the *body;* and, (b) in its most frequent usage, it is a description of syndromes that do *not* correlate with any organic condition, but are considered functional, mental, or spiritual disorders of the soul if and as you like (e.g., the functional psychoses, neuroses, and personality disorders). In the first usage, "mental illness" has the equivalent status of pneumonia or a broken leg — in short, it is no different from "physical illness." However, this is not the case in the second usage. When you use the term "mental illness" to describe functional disorders in which no underlying physical dysfunction exists, you are using the term as a *metaphor*, or *analogously*.

It is fair to say that most professionals and philosophers of science agree with Szasz (1961) regarding the "myth" of mental illness, and see the analogy between mental illness and physical illness as a poor one (Finkel, 1976): in too many significant ways, mental illnesses do not look like physical illnesses. This point cannot be ignored. We can group symptoms, such as "disconnected associations," "inappropriate emotions," "autism," and "ambivalence," and call them collectively, "schizophrenia," but that is just to *name it*, not designate something pathological "underneath."

So it is different from pneumonia; and you make different kinds of statements from this "named disorder." For example, a group of 100 individuals all diagnosed "schizophrenia" might also show a low incidence of "violent behaviors" in a given period of time; some labeled "schizophrenic" may "act out" violently, whereas many more will not; and we, the professionals, cannot tell with *certainty* which ones will or will not. We may make defendable speculations, but they are just that — speculations. To continue with the example, of the 100 schizophrenics, some will be "psychotic" (i.e., displaying hallucinations or delusions, or both, and showing gross impairment in perceiving and coping with reality) at any designated moment, but again, many will not. We cannot predict with certainty on the individual case level. Causal relations are simply not within the arena of forensic psychology.

The Royal Commission Report was coming to recognize that mental disease was neither "simple" nor *necessarily* exculpating. It may "relate" to the commission of a crime, or it may not; and the "relation" to the crime may be "graded"; so its bearing on the criminal act may be partial, a "contributory" but not the "specific cause," as Freud might have said. Here is their statement (*Durham,* Note 9):

> There is no *a priori* reason why every person suffering from any form of mental abnormality or disease, or from any particular kind of mental disease, should be treated by the law as not answerable for any criminal offense which he may commit, and be exempted from conviction and punishment. Mental abnormalities vary infi-

nitely in their nature and intensity and in their effects on the character and conduct of those who suffer from them. Where a person suffering from a mental abnormality commits a crime, there must always be some likelihood that the abnormality has played some part in the causation of the crime; and, generally speaking, the graver the abnormality, . . . the more probable it must be that there is a causal connection between them. But the closeness of this connection will be shown by the facts brought in evidence in individual cases and cannot be decided on the basis of any general medical principle. (p. 875)

The Durham rule protects a man from retribution for a crime that was not his doing (but the doing of his mental illness); however, it opens up a treacherous practical chasm: it demands a proof that cannot be provided. The professions that possess an ability to make educated speculations about the functional relationship between mind and action, the mental health profession being one, cannot determine what causality, if any, this mental illness–criminal action relationship may involve. This is precisely what Durham wants, as implied in the sentence, "He would still be responsible for his unlawful act if there was no causal connection between such mental abnormality and the act."

What the "expert" witness does is infer the causal relationship. His diagnosis of "mental illness" *implies* nonresponsibility. As Leifer (1964) states,

The point of this discussion is to show that mental disease is not an independent variable which is inversely related to the dependent variable of free choice, but it is *by definition* inversely related to it. The relationship is tautological and not factual. Since responsibility is *by definition* a function of intention, it logically follows that responsibility is definitionally related to the diagnosis of mental illness. Since the diagnosis of mental illness is considered a fact on which the psychiatrist is expert, then his conclusion that an act is the product of mental illness *logically* implies lack of intention and, thus, lack of responsibility. The determination of mental illness *logically* implies lack of intention determination similar to that with which the court is charged. . . . It is thus a logical error to consider mental disease to be a fact which is inversely correlated with intention, since mental disease is not a fact but is, like intention, ascribed on the basis of facts. (pp. 828–829)

CLOSING SUMMARY

Let us pause and reflect for a moment. The Courts seem to be marching to Justice Frankfurter's words, "I dare to believe that we ought not to rest content with the difficulty of finding an improvement in the M'Naghten Rules," but they seem to be following Psychology's tune regarding the nature of Psychological Man, the nature of "mental illness," and, as a consequence, the role, latitude, and exactitude of psychiatric testimony. The Court has not got its "steps-to-the music" right yet. It is time to call the tune into question, as well as the dancer's response. The Law, not wishing to appear dated and out of step, dancing to a state of psychological knowledge that went out years ago, keeps abreast of the "new time," "new view of man," and "new music," and changes to the "latest courtroom steps." The Law, acting very much the part of a woman blindfolded, gropes for the "Light" and finds Psychology, whom she sees as a "great advancement in medical science" and "as an enlightening influence on this subject." I wonder whether this Lady has not been "star-struck," blinded rather than enlightened, her reason and judgment dethroned rather than uplifted — but saddest of all — *had*. Perhaps she can plead in her own defense that it was temporary insanity.

Szasz (1970) sees the court's insanity, but thinks it comes from avoidance rather than from a love swoon (i.e., emotional insanity).

It must suffice to remark here that our age seems passionately devoted to *not* confronting problems of good and evil, and prefers, therefore, the rhetoric of medicine to the rhetoric of morals. It is as if modern judges had acquired the disability their predecessors had attributed to M'Naghten. M'Naghten, we are told, could not distinguish between right and wrong. Many judges, we may infer from their words and acts, prefer not to distinguish between right and wrong. They speak of mental health and sickness rather than of good and evil, and mete out the penalty of commitment rather than of imprisonment.

In the . . . case before the United States Court of Appeals for the Second Circuit, the moral problem was more difficult to evade than usual, but evaded it was. The defendant, Charles Freeman, had been convicted of selling heroin. He maintained that he was not guilty, by reason of insanity. In reversing the conviction, the court left open the possibility that under the new standards Freeman might be found insane. Yet, if ever there was a moral problem, this was it. The fundamental questions this case poses are whether it is good or bad to sell heroin, and whether or not such conduct should be prohibited by law. . . . Judge Kaufman's decision is significant precisely because it shifts the emphasis from the moral to the medical. In doing so, it exemplifies the "hysterical optimism" that, according to Richard Weaver, "will prevail until the world again admits the existence of tragedy, and it cannot admit the existence of tragedy until it again distinguishes between good and evil." (pp. 102–103)

This closing summary would be incomplete without a few words about the American Law Institute's Model Penal Code, which, in 1973, replaced the Durham rule in *United States* v. *Brawner*,[13] and Congress' proposed revision. The American Law Institute's model states that "a person is not responsible for criminal conduct if at the time of such conduct as a result of mental disease or defect he lacks substantial capacity to appreciate the criminality of his conduct as to conform to the requirements of law." The Law Institute format drops the term, "know," of M'Naghten for the more affective "appreciate." In this manner, the ambiguity of the term "knowledge" (discussed in M'Naghten section) dissipates somewhat as "understanding" is implied. Interpretive problems of "appreciate" will also occur, but the term is a less vague improvement. "Criminality of his conduct" seems to imply some awareness that he breached established law.

The revision proposed by Congress states that it is a "defense to a prosecution under any federal statute that the defendant, as a result of mental disease or defect, *lacked the state of mind required as an elmeent of the offense charged.* Mental disease or defect does not otherwise constitute a defense." (Italics mine.)

Whether the defendant lacked "substantial capacity" or the "state of mind required" is a judgment, an opinion, and not a scientifically determined fact. Psychology still cannot provide certainty here. There is however, something noticeably different here. The Law is no longer talking about sanity or insanity as an "either you have it or you do not" proposition, but is coming to recognize correlations, gradations, and "substantial" capacity: the capacity is not there or absent, but filled to a certain level.

This is leading us back to Isaac Ray's belief that reason is not completely obliterated in "mental disease," so some sense of right and wrong exists. I would agree with Ray, and would reverse the reversal of Durham: I would leave the burden of proving insanity to the defendant, and not put the burden on the government of proving sanity. This would no doubt make it harder to claim insanity and prove insanity, but this is as it should be, in my opinion.

If we assume some sense of right and wrong, and I would recommend this assumption in the vast majority of cases, then we should not exculpate completely for alleged mental illness. There are few exceptions to my recommendation. As I am writing this, I am sitting at my campsite in the George Washington National Forest in Virginia. I am looking out into the woods, sipping a Perrier and lime, and munching on chocolate fudge cookies. If a

---

[13] *Brawner* v. *U.S. supra*, Note 7, 986.

homo ferus trotted out of the woods, snatched my cookies and gulped my Perrier, I would pour him another and excuse his "offense." "He" I would exculpate. So one of my qualifying recommendations is to keep, the "wild beast" test but keep the mental health professional from deciding. (If the mental health professional wishes to be a modern-day Itard, and study, care for, and learn from the man–animal, then he has my blessing and best wishes.)

Also I would exculpate for someone who can medically document that his mental condition and behavior are caused by an underlying organic dysfunction for which he cannot insert self-control. So the defendant who demonstrates that certain stimuli "set off" electrical discharges in the brain that result in epileptic seizures and rage responses that he cannot stop once started, and who did not, by negligence (i.e., deliberately not taking one's medicine) or choice "set off" the chain of responses would be similarly exculpated. But this qualification would be invoked in very few cases.

What I have done is to limit severely the concept of "nondeterrable." Although I do not go as far as Szasz[14] (1970), I am in sympathy with his suggested direction.

For me these "mental conditions" are a mitigating, not exculpating factor, except for the above qualifications. Whether a man kills another with thoughtful premeditation or sudden passion, or because he is an alcoholic—drunk and driving—or is mentally unbalanced, does not, in my opinion, remove responsibility entirely. We do, in bifurcation of the trial into two phases, assess both *actus reus* (determining whether he committed the criminal act) and *mens rea* (determining the guilty mind of the accused). It is the *mens rea* part we are having such difficulty with. What does "evil mind" mean now? I am not denying "evil" or "tragedy" in this world, as Szasz suggests some do. Yet the yes-no, black-white demarcation line between Good and Evil seems more complex than that. In recognizing "mental illness" as complex and of varying types and degrees, the Royal Society suggests that the contribution of mental illness to the criminal behavior may be graded. Might we not ask, "Then should not the release from criminal responsibility be similarly graded?" This contrasts with the older notion of "all-or-none" insanity, expressed in the last paragraph of Durham (Note 9):

---

[14] Szasz (1970) states, "I do not believe that insanity should be an 'excusing condition' for crime. The insanity plea is abolished, or the sooner it disappears because of its dire consequences for the defendant, the better off we shall all be" (p. 109)

The legal and moral traditions of the western world require that those who, of their own free will and with evil intent (sometimes called *mens rea*), commit acts which violate the law, shall be criminally responsible for those acts. Our traditions also require that where such acts stem from and are the product of a mental disease or defect as those terms are used herein, moral blame shall not attach, and hence there will not be criminal responsibility. (p. 876)

Echoing the sentiments of Thomas Szasz and Chico Marx, I too, agree—that there is no insanity clause or defense—save when the brains do not work right or when the man-beast emerges from the woods. Yet there has been a lot of insanity on the question of insanity, much of it exacted by those whose "reason" and "judgment" were supposed to be expert; one expert testifies, technicalizes, and mystifies, placing himself in his own strait jacket; the other blindfolds herself and follows the tune; and Folly laughs.

POSTSCRIPT TO ACQUITTAL

So what happens when you are "acquitted by reason of insanity?" Szasz (1970) tells us what happened to Daniel M'Naghten:

> Since M'Naghten was acquitted, the reader might think that he was discharged by the court. Until 1843, this is what the word "acquittal" meant in the English language. But M'Naghten's "acquittal" was a precursor to that debauchment of language which, as Orwell taught us, is characteristic of modern bureaucratic societies. *De jure,* M'Naghten was acquitted; *de facto,* he was sentenced to life imprisonment in an insane asylum. He was confined at the Bethlehem Hospital until 1864, when he was transferred to the newly opened Broadmoor Institution for the Criminally Insane. M'Naghten died in Broadmoor in 1865, having been incarcerated for the last twenty-two years of his life. (p. 98)

Although this was M'Naghten's story and fate, what about the rest, the majority? Again, the voice is Szasz's (1970):

> There are two basic possibilities. One is that acquittal by reason of insanity is regarded as being the same as any other acquittal; the defendant walks out of the courtroom a free man. This is what happened to the fictional hero of Robert Traver's *Anatomy of a Murder.* It is what would have happend to Jack Ruby had Melvin Belli's defense strategy succeeded. This outcome is unusual and is becoming rarer every day.
>   The other course of action, which has been gaining ground rapidly in recent years, is to treat the individual acquitted by reason of insanity as a dangerously insane person from whom society

needs the utmost protection. Instead of walking out of the court-room a free man, such a defendant is forthwith transported to an insane asylum, where he remains until "cured" or until "no longer dangerous to himself and others." (p. 107)

So in the former his acquittal means freedom; in the latter, it means confinement—but this time a "therapeutic institutionalization." And the latter opinion is quite current, as Judge Kaufman voiced it in *United States* vs. *Freeman* (1966), and as Szasz comments:

> The American Law Institute rule embodies the same principle of automatic commitment. "Throughout our opinion," wrote Judge Kaufman, "we have not viewed the choice as one between imprisonment and immediate release. Rather, we believe the true choice to be between different forms of institutionalization—between the prison and the mental hospital. Underlying today's decision is our belief that treatment of the truly incompetent in mental institutions would better serve the interests of society as well as the defendant's."
>
> Consider what this means. The judge recognizes the defendant as mentally competent to stand trial; he allows him to enter a plea and defend himself as best he can, and he considers the defendant sane enough to be sentenced to the penitentiary if found guilty. But should the defendant be found "not guilty by reason of insanity," that verdict immediately transforms him into a "truly incompetent" person, whom the judge feels justified in committing to a mental hospital. "In former days," observed John Stuart Mill in his famous essay *On Liberty*, "when it was proposed to burn atheists, charitable people used to suggest putting them in the madhouse instead; it would be nothing surprising nowadays were we to see this done, and the doers applauding themselves, because, instead of persecuting for religion, they had adopted so humane and Christian a mode of treating these unfortunates, not without a silent satisfaction at their having thereby obtained their deserts." This was written when Freud was only three years old and when there was no "scientific psychiatry" to "illuminate" the problem of criminal responsibility (p. 108)

So more "word games" are being played: we go from someone "competent" to stand trial to a "truly incompetent" being, from "persecuting" to "treating," and we finally arrive at the last word transformation and stopping place, from "imprisonment" to "hospitalization."

Many, who view the "facts" and the "word games," find no difference between imprisonment and hospitalization. There are a number of such cases in Ennis' (1972) book that bears the title, *Prisoners of Psychiatry*. The courts have been more willing of late to scrutinize the facts of "hospitalization," "milieu therapy," and the like, to detect "euphemisms" that belie the true state of affairs; sometimes they have found both hospital and prison to be essentially equivalent forms of incarceration. Sometimes, as in Wyatt (Note 10), the hospital, if anything, seems more "cruel and inhumane" than prison. When Szasz (1970) looks at the facts, he does not see equivalence either: he finds hospitalization to be worse, only he terms it, "slavery disguised as therapy." The prisoner turned patient may find himself in a maximum security ward with less stimulation, space, and personal freedom than he would have had had he been in prison. When "mental disease" is acknowledged, he may lose more of his rights than a criminal would. As Szasz (1970) points out:

> Excepting death, involuntary psychiatric hospitalization imposes the most severe penalty that our legal system can inflict on a human being: namely, loss of liberty. The existence of psychiatric institutions that function as prisons, and of judicial sentences that are, in effect, indeterminate sentences to such prisons, is the backdrop against which all discussion of criminal responsibility must take place. This is especially true in jurisdictions where there is no death penalty. For what does it matter whether or not the accused was, at the time of the offense, "sane" and criminally responsible, or "insane" and criminally not responsible? (pp. 106–107)

When you meet Tom Szasz, especially after years of reading him and "hearing about" him, as I did, you peer into his soul and heart. There is bitterness there. But great courage, force, and intelligence. His spirit shines. His eyes twinkle (and that is especially important to me). He is sad and touched deeply by what *he sees*. And *see* he does; and he "calls" it unblinkingly. Some may think to excess or hyperbole, piercing the fabric not with a needle but with a howitzer, but all agree that Szasz's thoughts do pierce us. Let me use his words to summate:

> It is an idle hope that a scientific psychiatry will save us from moral problems and moral decisions. If we only let ourselves see with the eyes God gave us and with the courage that only we can give ourselves, we shall see legal psychiatry and involuntary mental hospitalization for what they are: a pseudo-medical system of social controls. . . .
>
> In the final analysis, the insanity plea and the insanity verdict, together with the prison sentences called "treatments" served in buildings called "hospitals," are all parts of the complex structure of institutional psychiatry, which, as I have tried to show, is slavery disguised as therapy. Those who value and wish to defend individual liberty can be satisfied with nothing less than the abolition of this crime against humanity. (Szasz, 1970, pp. 110–112)

FREDERICK LYNCH

The reader, at this point, seeing yet another case before him, may begin to question the sanity of the author. "Can't he stop his impulse to cite cases?" "Will it end?" The answer to both is yes. However, an indulgence is asked on behalf of the late Frederick C. Lynch, for his case imparts such important lessons regarding sanity, insanity, responsibility, and paternalism, that the telling of his tale may give us the best answer to the question, "Where will it all end?"

On November 6, 1959, Lynch walked into Municipal Court for the District of Columbia. He has been charged with passing bad checks. He drew two checks "in the amount of $50 each with knowledge that he did not have sufficient funds with the drawee bank for payment" (*Lynch* v. *Overholser*,[15] 1962). A plea of not guilty was recorded.

Then something *different* happened. The judge set a trial date, but commited Lynch to a hospital for a mental examination to determine his competency to stand trial. The original court record does not reveal the basis for the trial court's action. Did the judge suspect something? Did Lynch say something that might hint of mental illness? Did he act in some way that might cause suspicion? We do not know enough to judge the judge's judgment.

Almost one month later (Dec. 4, 1959), the assistant chief psychiatrist of the hospital reported that Lynch was then "of unsound mind, unable to adequately understand the charges and incapable of assisting counsel in his own defense." It was recommended that Lynch be given treatment at the hospital. The recommendation was accepted.

Twenty-four days later, the assistant chief of psychiatry wrote to the court that Lynch had "shown some improvement and at this time appears able to understand the charges against him, and to assist counsel in his own defense." It was also stated (the psychiatrist's opinion) that Lynch "was suffering from a mental disease, that is, a manic depressive psychosis, at the time of the crime charged," such that the crime "would be a product of this mental disease." This last statement is entirely gratuitous. It not only offers an opinion that was not asked for, but offers the Durham defense for the defendant — who had not asked for it.

In fact, Lynch repeatedly claimed *he did know* what he was doing.

The psychiatrist's report then returns *to what was asked,* and

---

[15] *Lynch* v. *Overholser,* 369 U. S. 705 (1962).

states that Lynch "appears to be in an early stage of recovery from manic depressive psychosis," but that it was "possible that he may have further lapses of judgment in the near future." He stated that it "would be advisable for him to have a period of further treatment in a psychiatric hospital."

The part of the report germane to that moment was his current functioning, not his functioning at the time of the act or at some future time. His current functioning was "recovering," so he could assist in his own defense. Lynch was brought to trial the next day in municipal court before a judge without a jury. Lynch, represented by counsel, *chose* to withdraw his earlier plea of not guilty, and to plead guilty. Lynch is saying, "I did it. I knew what I was doing. And did it." He may also be saying "I'd rather go to prison than get sent to a psychiatric hospital, so I wish to refuse treatment and take punishment." That was *his choise;* or so it seemed.

The trial judge refused to allow Lynch's change of plea. Now, a trial judge can refuse a plea. Said another way, a criminal defendant does not have an absolute right to have his guilty plea accepted by the court. But we have seen in Chapter 4 (*The Case for Controls* v. *The Right to Refuse Treatment*) the great dangers of overruling or undermining consent, and the consequences. So here was Lynch accepting responsibility for his act, willing to say "I knew it, did it, and I'm willing to face the punitive consequences for it," but the judge would not let him accept responsibility. The judge overruled Lynch's consent (to the guilty plea), and used the psychiatrist's "gratuitous" assertion of "mental illness at the time of the act" as the grounds. Undermined and overruled, Frederick Lynch was about to be caught as never before.

It may seem to some contradictory that a defendant found *competent* to stand trial can be, at the same moment, *not competent* to choose to plead guilty. In a way, Lynch was roped into the not guilty (by reason of insanity) plea. This may be another form of insanity; the court had not *seen* it this way; Lynch was coming to it.

The defense for this judicial practice (as the reader may have guessed by this time) is rooted in paternalism. The United States Court of Appeals[16] said, "Society has a stake in seeing to it that a defendant who needs hospital care does not go to prison and hence defendant and his counsel did not have absolute right to enter plea of guilty and preclude trial of issue of insanity."

So it was to be.

---

[16] *Overholser* v. *Lynch*, 288 F. 2d 388 (1961).

At the trial[17] one of the prosecution's witnesses, a physician representing the General Hospital's Psychiatric Division, testified, over petitioner's objection, that petitioner's crimes had been committed as a result of mental illness. Although petitioner never claimed that he had not been mentally responsible when the offenses were committed and presented no evidence to support an acquittal by reason of insanity, the trial judge concluded that petitioner was 'not guilty on the ground that he was insane at the time of the commission of the offense.' The court then ordered that petitioner be committed to Saint Elizabeth's Hospital as prescribed by D. C. Code 24-301 (d), which reads:

(d) If any person tried upon an indictment or information for an offense, or tried in the juvenile court of the District of Columbia for an offense, is acquitted solely on the ground that he was insane at the time of its commission, the court shall order such person to be confined in a hospital for the mentally ill.

A word or two about the enactment of D. C. Code 24-301 (d). It was quoted in Mr. Justice Harlan's opinion of the court in *Lynch* v. *Overholser* (Note 15) that "apprehension that Durham would result in a flood of acquittals by reason of insanity and fear that these defendants would be immediately set loose led to agitation for remedial legislation."

Fear must be acknowledged. Fear seems to have a deep and persistent motivation on courts, communities, and psyches; the seventeenth century's (real and imagined) fear of madness, of its contagion, corruption, or violent potential (or all of these), is with us *now*. The Newsweek (May 8, 1978) article, "Insanity on Trial," uses a "not guilty by reason of insanity" case, who was released in less than a year, and who then killed again, to highlight Chicagoans fear, outrage, and reactions to an insanity defense: "The Vanda case outrages Chicagoans who think the insanity defense is little more than a ploy used by killers, abetted by crafty defense lawyers and soft-hearted psychiatrists, to escape punishment" (p. 108).

However, if we recall Szasz's point in the previous section and the facts comparing the length of psychiatric hospitalization versus the length of prison sentences of a still earlier section, we know that the average insanity hospitalization is *longer,* most often, *indeterminate,* and often, *terminal.* I suspect Frederick Lynch knew that. He wanted to escape that fate. Not escape justice and punishment mind you (remember, he was willing to go to prison); but to escape indeterminate hospitalization.

---

[17] *Overholser* v. *Lynch,* 109 U.S. App. D.C. 404 (1959).

A *habeas corpus* proceeding, initiated by Lynch, resulted in his release, but the Court of Appeals reversed the district court, and Lynch was back in the hospital. The Court of Appeals reveals its "fear" and its paternalistic remedy of treatment: "We clearly (have) stated that imprisonment was *wrong* in the case of a mentally ill person, as well as a remedy which could not possibly secure the community against repetition of the offense" (Kittrie, 1971, p. 43). Unfortunately, neither prisons nor hospitals can *secure* "the community against repetition of the offense." But with "ordinary" criminals, it is enough that they have paid in time and in prison for their *past* action. No guarantees for the future. We, the community at large, live with this, as prisoners are released when their time is up. With "insane" criminals, however, there is a desire both to punish the past act while preventing future acts, and this is done by indefinite confinement — called "treatment." Frederick Lynch is feeling harassed. The psychiatric hospital is closing in around him, and he is being "secured" in ways he imagined only in bad dreams and nightmares. The nightmare is becoming real.

His case, and this story, reaches its last stop: the Supreme Court. The Court reversed the Court of Appeals, and found that D. C. Code 24-301(d) applies "only to a defendant acquitted on the ground of insanity who has affirmatively relied on a defense of insanity, and not to one who has maintained that he was mentally responsible when the alleged offense was committed" (p. 211). Justice Harlan noted that the District of Columbia statute flies in the face of Congress' attempt at safeguarding "those suspected of mental incapacity against improvident confinement." Judge Harlan noted how easy it was for Lynch to be "improvidently confined," and how Congress wished to safeguard against just that. "Hence if the accused denies that he is mentally ill, he is entitled to a judicial determination of his present mental state despite the hospital board's certification that he is of unsound mind. And it should be noted that the burden rests with the party seeking commitment to prove the accused is 'then of unsound mind.'"

Lynch never had a commitment hearing. With all the problems of commitment (see Chapter 3, section "'Due Reason, Inquiry, and Authority'—The Process of Confinement"), it offers the person *protections* (e.g., notice, right to counsel, opportunity to be heard and to cross-examine, etc.) that Lynch never had.

Lynch was undermined. In football, he was blind-sided, while in judicial circles, one court tells another that its sight is blinded and its judgment is in error.

Courts speak through their dissents, as well as their opinions. Let us look selectively at Mr. Justice Clark's dissent in Lynch. Clark worries that Lynch was mentally ill (a) at the time of the act, (b) at the time of his plea (since Clark notes Lynch "made no attempt to appeal from the refusal of the court to accept his guilty plea"), (c) for the next six months (since Clark notes that Lynch did not file for habeas corpus for some six months, six months of treatment, to Clark, so Judge Clark infers that Lynch may not have been sane enough to file — an inference that does not give Lynch the benefit of doubt), (d) currently (since "the last doctor's report in the record shows him to be suffering from a manic depressive psychosis from which though he 'appears to be in an early stage of recovery' it is 'possible that he may have further lapses' ") and (e) in the future. ("It further states that it 'would be advisable for him to have a period of further treatment in a psychiatric hospital.' The order today risks bringing that to an end.").

Clark is voicing the community's fear and worry, and its desire for security. He wrote: "But insane offenders are no less a menace to society for being held irresponsible, and reluctance to impose blame on such individuals does not require their release. The community has an interest in protecting the public from antisocial acts whether committed by sane or by insane persons" (p. 223). The reader may be thinking that Clark had in mind "murderers and the like," not "bad check writers." (Bad check writers get one year, maximum — maybe suspended sentence.) However, here is what Clark said: "We have long recognized that persons who because of mental illness are dangerous to themselves or to others may be restrained against their will in the interest of public safety and to seek their rehabilitation, even if they have done nothing proscribed by the criminal law. The insane who *have committed acts otherwise criminal are a still greater object of concern,* as they have demonstrated *their risk to society*" (p. 223). (Italics mine.)

Judge Clark is not seeing Lynch as a "bad check writer," but as a risk.

Lynch, a "risk to society"? We will never know. Frederick Lynch's last act brought his "improvident confinement" and this story to an end. He opened the story, and closed it. As lawyers are wont to say, he made the case moot — but not the *point*.

Frederick Lynch punned himself to death. He lynched himself.

6

I come to the last chapter feeling like Goethe's one treadle which throws a thousand threads hither and thither; now it is time to knit those threads together.

We have touched upon many areas: the techniques of therapy, the process of confinement, contractual therapy, and involuntary treatment; questions of paternalism, ethics, consent, competency, and the right to refuse treatment; and insanity, in citizens, courts, communities, and in "benefactors" and "beneficiaries." If there is a signal thread that weaves these issues together, perhaps we would not err too greatly if we call that supportive threat "benevolence," and agree to use the term (Merriam-Webster, 1971, p. 80) in the following way: "*n* 1: disposition to do good 2a: an act of kindness b: a generous gift." We now come to the central underlying question: "What are the limits of benevolence?" David Rothman, in a marvelous book entitled *Doing Good: The Limits of Benevolence* (Gaylin, Glasser, Marcus, & Rothman, 1978), asks the question this way: "Where should the authority of the caretaker leave off and the rights of the cared-for begin?" (pp. xi–xii)

We are about to take a close look at our acts of kindness, looking generous gifts in the mouth and gift givers in the eye. For to put it succinctly, and in Rothman's words, "We recognized that a claim once considered to be of the most virtuous sort, the claim to be acting benevolently, had now become — to understate the point — suspect: if the last refuge of the scoundrel was once patriotism, it now appeared to be the activity of 'doing good' for others, acting in the best interest of someone else" (p. x).

A Closing Note: Lessons of History, Mythology, and Psychology A Divine Comedy — Balancing Justice and Mercy

For me, as a psychologist and parent, with a child about me and my childlike side within me, some of the toughest questions to face concern balancing my giving against my not giving, their needs against their rights, my needs against my limitations, and my paternalism against my ethics. I want to do *good*, yet I want to do *right*. How then, do I balance justice and mercy?

When consciously confronting questions that rack me personally and psychically, my unconscious often comes to the rescue in the form of an image – a transpersonal mythologm that transports me beyond the personal, to the mythic. The image that came to me, in two different forms, was that of the goddess, Justice. There she was, standing before me as she stands outside many a courthouse, beautiful and blindfolded, holding the tipped scales of justice in her hand. As a mythic figure she is Wisdom: called Sophia, Athena, Eve, Sakti, the Muse, or the Shekhinah, she represents the Eternal Female in one of her aspects; as a personal, psychic figure, she is my feminine side, my anima and shadow, whom I seek to see and know. The image came in two forms. The second form of the goddess of Justice came from a Tarot card, number XI of the major arcana. The key differences between these two images were (a) in the Tarot image, Justice does not have on a blindfold, but sees, and (b) in the Tarot image, the scales are balanced, rather than tipped (Gray, 1970). There are many other differences of course, but these two struck and stuck with me. But why these differences? Why the blindfold? What does it mean? Not blindness, but blindfolded. Capable of seeing, but choosing not to see. Something about conscious and 149 unconscious knowledge, balance and imbalance stuck with me. I mused on and on. Readers (and fellow psychologists) might consider my obsessive ruminations "esoteric," if they were being benevolent, or "diagnostically significant," in less generous, more clinical, moments. But I must confess that I was caught by the incongruity and image, and chose to pursue it. Here is where it took me.

The *Kabbalah.* It means "receiving" – receiving Wisdom. And if ever I needed to receive Wisdom, now was the time. So, to these writings of Jewish mysticism (Scholem, 1961) I went, seeking Divine guidance for my current imbalance. What I found, in one of my sources (Singer, 1977), was a Talmudic analogy, which is quite apropos to this moment:

> First, the Holy One, Blessed be He, tried to create the world according to the measure of mercy [grace] but it fell apart. Then he tried to create it according to the measure of justice [*din,* judgment] but that too fell apart. What did he do? He took an equal measure of mercy and mixed it with an equal measure of justice, and the result was our world. (p. 154)

It would seem, then, that the Holy One, too, had problems holding it together – in balance. It was comforting to be in such good company. However, the Holy One eventually got it right, and I was a long way off. I did get some compassion for our human predicament out of this Talmudic tale, as well as confirmation that these personal, professional, and historical difficulties of balance were "toughies." I also received guidance, letting the myth be my guide. I went back to the Tarot for a reading.

One of the images that repeated itself in several of the major cards was that of a figure seated between two pillars (Justice, card XI; the Hierophant, card V; and the High Priestess, card II). The two pillars are described in the following quote (Gray, 1970):

> The High Priestess is seated between two pillars from the Temple of Solomon – the black pillar of Boaz representing the negative life force, and the white one, Jachin, the positive life force.
>
> Thomas Troward, in his book *The Hidden Power,* has this to say about the two pillars before the temple: "They contain the key to the entire Bible and to the whole order of Nature, and as emblems of the two great principles that are the pillars of the universe, they fitly stood at the threshold of that temple which was designed to symbolise all the mysteries of Being."

Shuffling back to the Kabbalah, we have those two pillars again, representing parts of the *Sefiroth,* ten aspects of the Divinity and ten stages of the inner world that metaphorically retell the story of Genesis – the Creation – by which the *En Sof* (the "limitless" or "boundless" which is everywhere and nowhere – no thing) emanates, and descends from the inmost recesses down to His revelation. Two of these ten *Sefiroth*, *Hokmah* and *Binah*, represent "wisdom" and "intelligence," the "head" and the "heart," the "masculine" and the "feminine." These pillars represent polarities, dualities that are paradoxically contained in the One. Under these two are *Gevurah*, judgment or "sternness," and *Hesed*, "mercy" or "love."

To summarize, we see the portrayal in cards, life, and myth of "apparent" opposites: wisdom–understanding, head–heart, positive–negative, reason–unreason, sternness–love, male–female, conscious–unconscious, and Justice–Mercy. We also see, from the Talmudic analogy of balance and from historical examples of imbalances and treatment failures, that Justice and Mercy must somehow "go together," but seldom do. "*Justice* and *Mercy*, in the sefirothic schema, represent feminine and masculine elements, respectively, and so it is clear that without a harmonious balance between the two, the world could not have been created" (Singer, 1977, p. 154). Yet, in the world of men, with its divisions, reason–madness nexus, and alternations between periods of sternness (e.g., the expulsion of madness aboard ships of fools, or the practice of confinement) and mercy (e.g., moral treatment), we have not been able to create a harmonious balance. *Hokmah* and *Binah*, which have been called the "two friends who never part" (Singer, 1977, p. 158), seem to be doing much better *above* the firmament than *below*. Unfortunately, history and reality (ours) have yet to match the mythic union of *Justice* and *Mercy*.

I wish to step out of the mythic and back into our world, back to the question and limits of benevolence. I will let the mythic image percolate, and bubble through at timely points. For now, however, it recedes to its collective unconscious source, as I proceed.

IN THE BEGINNING

Willard Gaylin, a psychoanalyst, tells us, in his article entitled "In the Beginning: Helpless and Dependent" (Gaylin, Glasser, Marcus, & Rothman, 1978), that we all go through an extended period of dependency, and that it is crucial for the development of a person that there be someone who loves, cares, and gives. As he states: "We are caring people, despite the fact that it may be fashionable now to deny it . . . we respond not only to the child, but to the childlike; we respond to the helpless, whether animal or human" (p. 20). Gaylin tells us that our parentalism and caring is part of our nature as *Homo sapiens*. He writes:

> Caring—that is, the protective, parental, tender aspects of loving —is a part of relationship among peers, child to parent, friend to friend, lover to lover, person to animal. The parent–child aspect of caring is only the essential paradigm whose presence is necessary for the diffusion of this human quality into the other relational aspects of life. The linkages between being cared for and caring for others are crucial to remember. (p. 33)

Yet in our current time,

> It is fashionable . . . to view paternalism and benevolence as obscene terms. The reformers of the past are often ridiculed for failures to achieve their ends. Worse, their intentions are suggested to be motivated by unconscious self-serving. "Unconscious motives" are dirty words best left to the privacy of the psychoanalytic retreat. Judge not that ye be not judged. I have little faith in the eventual success of the best-intended of our current laborers in their efforts for equity and justice. Still I revere their intentions and their effort.
> There will always be the need for parental compassion; at the same time, there will always be the need for vigilance in recognizing the limitations of institutions of government as surrogate parents. Nonetheless, it is not parentalism that is the crime, it is what is passed off for parentalism. (p. 32)

Gaylin is seeing the historical winds shifting again: where, in past years, the progressive and humanistic forces were in the ascendant (Robinson, 1973; Rothman, 1978), we now seem to be witnessing an ebb tide, if not a full-scale retreat from paternalism and benevolence. As Rothman said, "The wisdom of the fathers seems, though perhaps mistakenly, wrongheaded to the sons" (p. xiii).

Gaylin worries, as Mercy retreats before the winds of Justice and as parent and therapist are replaced by lawyers, that we may again miss the boat.

Yet few would deny that paternalism has run amuck, and that its honorable intent has spawned some dishonorable practices. How has this happened? Ira Glasser, a lawyer, takes up this question in his article entitled "Prisoners of Benevolence: Power versus Liberty in the Welfare State" (Gaylin, Glasser, Marcus, & Rothman, 1978). Glasser takes a harsher view of man than Gaylin; where Gaylin sees caring people, Glasser sees sharks, and turns to our forebearers and their document, the Bill of Rights, to justify his point. He asserts that our ancestors were less innocent regarding our "benevolence;" for they also saw man's other side, his "shadow," if you permit me a Jungian intrusion, an "aggressiveness," that uses power to trespass and seeks dominion; and therefore a counterpower, motivated by fear, needed to be asserted to limit "the endlessly propulsive tendency" of power. Never mind that the power is being used by parents, those who posture as parents, or so-called parent surrogates; let the child beware, and be less innocent. That is why it did not surprise our forebearers that Jefferson, the architect and apostle of liberty, would, *when president,* be much less the civil libertarian. Glasser quotes a passage from Levy's work, "Jefferson and Civil Liberties: The Darker Side," which goes as follows:

> Jefferson at one time or another supported loyalty oaths; countenanced internment camps for political suspects; drafted a bill of attainder; urged prosecutions for seditious libel; trampled on the Fourth Amendment; condoned military despotism; used the army to enforce laws in time of peace; censored reading; chose professors for their political opinions; and endorsed the doctrine that the means, however, odious, were justified by the ends. . . . Jefferson's lapses were in large part natural and to be expected. They "did not result from hypocrisy or meanness of spirit," but rather derived, in part, from the fact that many circumstances seemed to Jefferson to require the sacrifice of his libertarian ideals for "larger" and more compelling governmental ends. (p. 105)

So just because we say we are "doing good," providing treatment and therapy, or offering social services does not mean that that is the whole story. Again, a quote from Glasser:

> This undifferentiated view of social services . . . tended to blind liberals to certain unintended consequences of their good works. Because their motives were benevolent, their ends good, and their purpose caring, *they assumed the posture of parents* toward the recipients of their largesse. They failed utterly to resist the impulse toward paternalism, which in another context Bernard Bailyn called "the endlessly propulsive tendency" of power to expand itself and establish *dominion* over people's lives. They eagerly embraced such dominion and persuaded themselves that by doing so they were helping the helpless. Dominion became legitimate: those who managed social services — not infrequently liberals themselves — came to enjoy a degree of discretionary power over their clients that normally only parents are allowed over their children. As a result, they infantilized those they intended to help, and denied them their rights. (p. 107)

Glasser's conclusion and recommendation are the following:

> It is not that benevolence is itself mischievous or cynically to be regarded with mistrust. It is not benevolence we should abandon, but rather the naive faith that benevolence can mitigate the mis-

chievousness of power so feared by those who wrote our Bill of Rights. We have traditionally been seduced into supposing that because they represented charity, service professionals could speak for the best interests of their clients. By now we should know better. (p. 123)

THEIR BROTHERS' KEEPERS

Something happens when men act benevolently,[1] that, in the eyes of history and hindsight, makes us wince. What starts out to be benevolent action or paternalism in its most caring form comes out perverted and distorted. So as Gaylin (1978) reminds us, it is not paternalism per se, but what passes for paternalism that is the problem. There is a second part to this perversion of benevolence process: not only is the action suspect, but the "benevolent" actor seems to have *no suspicion* that anything is wrong. As Glasser notes, there is a naive faith in the "doer of good." I translate "naive faith" into tunnel vision or blindness (or both) and invoke more psychological terms that traditionally deal with naive, "unconscious" processes, such as "denial," "repression," and "projection" in order to shed some light.

Steven Marcus, in his essay "Their Brothers' Keepers: An Episode from English History" (Gaylin, Glasser, Marcus, & Rothman, 1978), asks the question:

"How is it, we must continue to ask, that good people — decent, upright, and well-meaning citizens — can contrive, when they act on behalf of others and in the name of some higher principle or of some benign interest, to behave so harshly, coercively, and callously, so at odds with what they understand to be their good intentions" (p. 42). Marcus goes on to show, by examining the Poor Laws in England, particularly a paternalistic apparently liberal law change that offered relief to the "able-bodied poor," introduced in 1795. This regulation introduced the idea of a "right to live," and, to quote another historian, "No measure was ever more universally popular. Parents were free of the care of their children, and children were no longer dependent upon parents; employers could reduce wages at will, and workers were safe from hunger whether they were busy or slack; humanitarians applauded the measure as an act of mercy even though not of justice and the selfish gladly consoled themselves with the thought that though it was merciful at least it was not liberal" (p. 48). Marcus (1978) comments:

---

[1] At this juncture, I am using the terms "benevolence," "paternalism," and "parentalism" quite interchangeably.

A monster had been created. A long-term demoralization set in upon a countryside that was already demoralized. However long it took, the ordinary man was sooner or later pushed onto relief, and the countryside as a whole was moving toward pauperization and loss of self-respect. The freeborn Englishman's right to protection had been transformed into mass dependency, which, at the moment, seemed preferable to the rootless independence of a free wage laborer in an open market. And paradoxically, this preference led to the human degradation that is historically inseparable from the English experience of early capitalism in both town and country. (p. 48)

It seems that what started out as a merciful act, a paternalistic law that extended the benevolent hand of the parent–government (with a shilling or two enclosed) to the freeborn, quickly turned independent men into dependents; in Gaylin's terms, those who were not "intrinsically dependent" (i.e., those "so physically, mentally, or emotionally handicapped that they are incapable of taking care of themselves, such as some of the mentally ill, mentally retarded, crippled, or senile") were turned into "extrinsically dependent" (i.e., those "made dependent by artifacts of our culture").

This is the indignity and infantilization that makes us wince and turn our eyes. "It is an indignity for an adult who has no intrinsic needs for care and maintenance to be reduced to the level of a child — with all the concomitant humiliations — because of a social system that deprives him of the rites of passage into maturity. We have seen how love, kindness, and caring first require self-pride and self-love. It is crucial that one who is capable be allowed to see oneself as adult. If we can find ways to eliminate the category of the extrinsically dependent, it is we who will benefit (Gaylin, 1978, p. 30).

Returning, for a moment, to the Poor Law in England and its drastic consequences, Malthus proposed a draconian solution: public relief did no good and had to be withheld; the poor must defend themselves; "nature" must be reintroduced into society, and allowed to take its course; the poor, or those who survived the mass deaths, would learn the virtues of self-dependence and self-sustainment; and, as a clergyman himself, Malthus proposed sermons to the dependent poor on moral and marital restraint. As Marcus (1978) notes, "Malthus had his followers, but the harshness of this proposal was too much even for those harsh times" (p. 52).

If the loving hand of Mercy created a mess, then the stern hand of Malthus and Justice would clean it up. Flip-flop. Yet in America, when Dorothea Lynde Dix became aware and then appalled by the neglect of the mentally ill, she mercifully suggested that these unfortunates be made "wards of the nation" (Finkel, 1976). Flop-flip.

Regarding Justice and Mercy, historical hegemony of one, then the other, seems to be the pattern. When one is in the ascendant while the other is on vacation, rather than hegemony giving way to that mythical marriage and harmony of the two in one, we get extremes of sternness or love, leading to neglect or infantilization. Marcus (1978) summarizes, in the following passage:

> So I imagine what I am saying — and I imagine what I have learned — is that we can degrade people by caring for them; and we can degrade them by not caring for them; and in matters such as these there are neither simple answers nor simple solutions. (pp. 65–66.)

BONDAGE, FALSE PROPHETS, AND AN EXODUS

Let us return to the "reason-madness nexus," as Foucault (1973) called it, where, in the classical period, men of reason placed their mad brethren on the other side of bars under the eyes of a reason that no longer felt any relation to it and that would not compromise itself by too close a resemblance. Madness had become a thing to look at: no longer a monster inside oneself, but an animal with strange mechanisms, a bestiality from which man had long since been suppressed."

When men of reason placed their brothers in bondage, in houses of confinement, the brotherhood was shattering. The madman would no longer be just our foolish, dark, unreasonable, unconscious side; the light of reason refused to see kinship and connection; consciousness was split, and *our* "shadow" became *the* "Other." He is now another, who becomes an object, a symbol, which we begin to "invest" with our excesses — our best and worst intentions. Fears, unconscious though they be — get projected into the Other, and, as a result, we greatly overpredict his dangerousness; with projections unrecognized, we can then justify to ourselves stronger, more coercive actions; and we can call those actions "treatment." Pity and caring still exist, since the kinship can be denied but not severed; yet the caring comes out twisted, overdone and overlayed with unrecognized determinants. As Rothman (1978) says, "Some paradox in our nature leads us, once we have made our fellow men the objects of our enlightened interest, to go on to make them the objects of our pity, then of our wisdom, ultimately of our coercion" (p. 72).

Whether by fear or care, the two roads lead to the same coercive path.

The new element in this script is the physician, the emissary to that "other world" of madness (Foucault, 1973). If the physician, or one of his modern heirs, the psychiatrist, psychologist, or mental health professional, was to cross the nexus and silence and reestablish the primordial harmony, he must have taken a wrong turn somewhere. No march out of bondage resulted – no exodus – only silence.

Justice, however, could put on the blindfold, assuring herself that the madmen were in good hands – being *treated* by an expert – the caring physician; and she has kept the blindfold on, being blind and enchanted by the words and promises of the psychological expert. Like a distorted and reversed form of the myth of Amor and Psyche, the goddess of Justice, in darkness, follows her mortal psyche through his theories of insanity, trying to keep pace with the "new time" and the "new steps." I believe the goddess has faltered, been led astray, and had. My recommendation is that the goddess of Justice take off her blindfold, for at least as long as it takes to recognize that the expert witness who sits in the witness seat and sits on the scales of justice, tips those scales by virtue of his weight, rather than by his wisdom. She would do well to unload this excess baggage.

I wrote earlier in this work, "Let the courts beware! Over the last 100 years, the court and the mental health profession have courted one another, for different reasons, each looking to the other for answers and respectability that were not coming from within. Before the wedding is consummated, and before the inevitable 'morning after' occurs, we ought to now face honestly whether the promise made can be kept. For judgments based on unreliable practices may promise certainty, only to give way to doubt and illusion the morning after. My prenuptial advice is twofold, sincere, but somewhat trite: for the groom, the paternalistic professinal, 'demonstrate reliability before making vows'; for the blindfolded bride, the court, 'look out.' "

Well, it seems we have arrived at the inevitable "morning after." One might ask, "Can her virtue be saved?" "Or repaired?" All need not be lost; gain often emerges out of apparent loss. Experience is a great teacher, if we do not remain blind to its lessons. The goddess has been burnt, yes. In Amor and Psyche, it was he who was burnt by her spilling of the oil; yet the spilling of the oil brought light to darkness and brought a new consciousness to a relationship that was incomplete, to say the least. Perhaps the myth will provide us the way out, if not the moral.

If Justice removes her blindfold, she will come to see what

Chief Justice Burger saw in 1964, that "psychology is, at best, an infant among the family of science, . . . and that psychiatrists and psychologists may be claiming too much in relation to what they really understand about the human personality and human behavior." And if she reads the literature on predicting dangerousness, she will realize that no one can. She wed under the presumption of his expertise. As I read it, the lady has grounds for an annulment. Her exodus from this ill-conceived marriage, coupled with his exodus from the courtroom, would go a long way toward bringing Psychology and Justice to a more balanced, and proper, relationship.

THE CASE FOR COMPASSION

"Blowing the whistle" on the unwholesome relationship between courts and mental health professionals, and the unfair practices that result, has been by the lawyers. If the seventeenth century delegated the physician as emissary to the madman, the last half of the twentieth century has seen the lawyers come to fill that role. The dialogue between reason and madness that had lapsed into silence at the end of the eighteenth century has resumed, full scale. The alleged madman now has a mouthpiece, an advocate, whose orientation changes from "doing good" to "doing right." Where the well-meaning parent (be he parent, state, court, or mental health professional) focuses on the person's *needs* and desires to promote equality among all, the legal advocate focuses on the person's *rights* and seeks to protect liberty.

A benevolent relationship, that is, "we are trying to do good for you," has given way to an adversarial relationship. Some find this turn of events saddening; others feel it represents an emergence out of an age of innocence. We have been innocent, in a way: innocent in assuming a *congruence of interest* between parent and child. But this innocence is rooted in the normal parent-child relationship. As Gaylin (1978) writes:

> The helpless child, of course, cannot speak for himself, and we must trust that identity of interest bound in nature that generally insures the compassionate concern of the parent for child. We grant, therefore, great power in this relationship not just because the child is the ultimate responsibility of the parent but because we are inclined to trust the general concern of the parent.
>
> It is obvious, however, that the relation of a mother to a child may differ from that of the father and will surely differ from that of the brother or sister or aunt or uncle or second cousin once removed. As we move farther and farther away from our original

paradigm we rightfully trust less the natural bonds of affection that tie the caretaker to the dependent. We are more inclined to legalistically hedge the power of the surrogate, and we would be wise to assume an increasing divergence between the interests of the helpless and the self-interest of the strong. The parent of a healthy six-month-old child simply does not bear the same relation to that child that an estranged son-in-law does to the senile, wealthy old lady to whom he is the next of kin.

When we move farther from the concept of next of kin to vesting authority in a social or political institution, our original paradigm becomes stretched quite thin. No social institution, regardless of how benevolent or paternalistic, can ever replicate the parent-to-child symbiosis." (pp. 27–28).

We used to assume a harmony of interest. So juvenile courts and probation officers assumed the privileges of parents to restrain their child. It did not work. Restraints did not hold. What started out as wholesome parental restraints turned unwholesome, and then coercive. "To claim to act for the purpose of benevolence was once sufficient to legitimatize a program; at this moment it is certain to create suspicion" (Rothman, 1978, p. 82). The suspicion now extends back to the original parent–child bond. To quote Rothman:

Whereas once it was assumed that parents would invariably act in the best interests of the child, even in the midst of divorce proceedings, now it seems the better part of wisdom to have children represented by their own attorney. Indeed, before parents can commit their child to a mental hospital, it is becoming obligatory that the child be represented by an attorney.

In effect, reform policy presupposes a conflict of interests among these parties, conflicts which before were never admitted to or adknowledged. . . . The very notion of a harmony of interests seems deceptive and mischievous. (pp. 86–87)

So we now have the adversarial movement — and confrontation; the false harmony of interests has given way. When it comes to the alleged mentally ill — or the weak, helpless, or disenfranchised — for that matter, we no longer know who is speaking for whom. Parental claims and documented kinship no longer mean congruence of interest. How then, is the goddess of Justice to tell what is in the person's best interest? How is she to see the truth?

Now, the image of the blindfold returns, as does the writings of the Kabbalah. In the latter, that which balances *Hokmah* and *Binah*, wisdom and intelligence, is *Kether*, the crown. *Kether*, which represents compassion, holds the two pillars, *Hokmah* and *Binah*, together: it idealizes the union of the two into One. So if there is any way to harmonize and balance Justice and Mercy, we would likely find it through compassion. Yet the *Kether* represents the highest point, where the hitherto unmanifest becomes knowable to us, and where the manifest passes into the unknown. My suggestion, at this point, may seem paradoxical, if not contradictory, in light of what I have recommended previously; now, I urge the goddess of Justice to put on her blindfold. For Divine Wisdom "lies beyond the horizon of human experience," and if she is going to *see* it, better she is not distracted by our dim lights.

So perhaps the two images of Justice, blindfolded and seeing, compliment and complete one another. Her seeing in the here and now, when we go astray and claim divine foresight and expertise; and *seeing* that higher wisdom, when we are groping and blind.

I am not satisfied, however. Myths seems to resolve themselves more clearly than earthly messes. The myth's solution can not be mine; for my eyes do not get above the firmament, veiled or not. And so it is with courts, judges, and juries, plaintiffs, defendants, psychiatrists, and psychologists, all who bear the mark of mortality. What are we to do when we can not *see* beyond?

I say, "then listen." Listen to the dependent one and his advocate. If he needs our help, let him ask. That is a first step in assuming responsibility. The difference between the public welfare state and the therapeutic state (Kittrie, 1971) is that the former is voluntary, whereas the latter is involuntary. Let us continue to give, and be merciful. As Gaylin (1978) says, "When we neglect the weak and helpless, the disenfranchised and disadvantaged, we betray our loving nature and endanger the social future that depends on our caring" (pp. 34–35); but let us hear their terms, and see our excesses. As Marcus (1978) concludes, "Dependents, precisely because they are dependent and often unable to help themselves, deserve more than others to be protected from the unintended consequences of our benevolence and the incalculable consequences of our social good will" (p. 66).

So in trying to do the most good, let us also remember to do the least harm. Navigating between the excesses of neglect and benevolence has not been easy, historically. The channel markers of Divine Wisdom or Aristotle's Golden Mean have been difficult to see. Perhaps greater compassion for our own predicament will offer us some needed solace; yet it is Wisdom we yearn for; and that seems to come from a growing consciousness – one that sees undistortedly and equally into regions of light and dark, conscious and unconscious, weighing its own actions against its intentions, and, while not resting – for there is more to do – can at least pause and say, "It is good."

THE DISSOLUTION OF TRANSFERENCE

Dear Dickensian Character:

To you, my created, hypothetical character of Chapter 2, I owe an answer. In Chapter 2 I left you hanging out, and then in Chapter 3, hanging on for dear life as you were being hauled away "for your own good." You shouted out to me, the mental health professional, and any listener or reader still within earshot or eyeshot, to explain "Why?!" . . . I remained silent. In Chapter 4, as you were losing control and consent, and as a result, your brain, mind, and being were in danger of violation in the name of greater freedom, you again shouted for explanation. In Chapter 5, we testified expertly that you were insane, defended you innocence by reason of insanity, whether you liked it or not, and you hung your head in silence.

This letter is my belated answer. It took me until Chapter 6 to put it together. The letter is also going public. "Sorry" for this violation of confidentiality, but we never did have a therapeutic contract. And anyway, I have to close this book and story about therapy and ethics, and the readership is expecting something. So to all who read my last chapter, letter, and testament, I am proposing willfully a dissolution of transference — with love.

Here are the specifics. I promise to leave you alone on your sidewalk spot; if you want to mumble or shout to the heavens, fine; you might even put in a good word for me, if the spirit moves you. But I will not move you.

There is a condition, though. Do not harm me or anyone else! I will support your freedom, but do not infringe on mine. If you do, all deals are off. For I have my copy of the Constitution too, and J.S. Mill as well, and I intend to use both to ensure my safety.

If you do me no harm, however, I will not act in your best interests. I will not exercise paternalism over your objections, no matter how sure and certain I feel. Your actions and life may bring me some psychic pain, but that is what I and the community of reasonable men need to bear for our paternalism.

You know, my Dickensian friend, I have fresh appreciation of you. I have just been reading Steven Marcus (1978), who cites an early poem by Wordsworth, "The Old Cumberland Beggar," that could have been about you. If we exchange beggar for allegedly mentally ill, and substitute rural for an urban setting, it might fit:

"Him from my childhood have I known; and then
He was so old, he seems not older now;
He travels on, a solitary man."

The beggar, alone, ancient, barely conscious, wanders on his end-
less round in the community. People know him and give him food,
sometimes alms or coins. He is not useless, Wordsworth insists; he
is not a nuisance. He is part of the habitual world of the community, and he even brings out feelings of kindliness and common
obligation in all who see him regularly. He is a "silent monitor" to
all who know him, and he is not to be pitied. For though he is
dependent, there is also something independent about him as well.
He is alone, but not in the way the English poor would be alone
some forty years later. Wordsworth moves his poem toward its
conclusion with the following lines:

"Then let him pass, a blessing on his head!
And, long as he can wander, let him breathe
The freshness of the valleys; let his blood
Struggle with frosty air and winter snows;
And let the chartered wind that sweeps the heath
Beat his grey locks against this withered face.
Reverence the hope whose vital anxiousness
Gives the last human interest to his heart.
May never HOUSE, misnamed of INDUSTRY,
Make him a captive! — for that pent-up din,
Those life-consuming sounds that clog the air,
Be his the natural silence of old age!
Let him be free of mountain solitudes;
And have around him, whether heard or not,
The pleasant melody of woodland birds.
Few are his pleasures: if his eyes have now
Been doomed so long to settle upon earth
That not without some effort they behold
The countenance of the horizontal sun,
Rising or setting, let the light at least
Find a free entrance to their languid orbs.
And let him, where and when he will, sit down
Beneath the trees, or on a grassy bank
Of highway side, and with the little birds
Share his chance-gathered meal; and, finally,
As in the eye of Nature he has lived,
So in the eye of Nature let him die!"

(pp. 55–57)

So friend, if someone tries to commit you, and it is not voluntary, I suggest that you get a lawyer, and support your right to
counsel as well as your right to notice, an opportunity to be heard
and cross-examine, protection against self-incrimination, and
proof beyond a reasonable doubt. I would support making civil

proceedings and safeguards as rigorous and protecting as in criminal proceedings. If I am called to testify, I will say what I know. But I will admit to not being an expert. I will admit that my, and my fellow professionals' diagnostic accuracy, is not high, be it for distinguishing sane from insane or for reliably separating shades of madness. I will also admit that my predictions of dangerousness are likely to be unlikely and overinflated. And I will suggest, if my expert opinion still allows me to make suggestions, that the court would be wise to take my suggestions with equal grains of salt and skepticism.

Although I will support your rights in civil commitment proceedings, I will not support you financially. I would recommend that tax dollars not go to your support, and that support be entrusted to you, as mine is to me. If you wish to take up Wordsworth's beggar's bowl, fine; a noble occupation; may Christian charity be kind to you. I may contribute myself, depending on my bank balance or mood — no guarantees, however. We have no contract and obligation.

If you, unfortunately, do become a resident of a psychiatric hospital (this is implying that you did not want to take up residence in that "condemnminium") and if you want my help in getting treatment and out, I will see what I can do, but you see what you have to do — no contract, no obligation.

If someone wishes to explore your brain with microelectrodes, or whatever else happens to be current, I would support your right to refuse — if you do not want the "treatment."

By the way, if you happen to be hauled into court for an *action* of yours that violates the law, and you want to plead "insane," or "innocent by reason of insanity," I promise I *will not* help you. I do not buy it. You can try to sell it to your peers, the jury. I support your right to make the case for extenuating, maddening circumstances, but not for exculpation. And I promise, if you do not want to claim insanity, I will not hang you with it.

That is where I stand. If you ever get tired of sidewalks, want to put some change in your life and are thinking about therapy, stop by. If *you* like, we can chat; see if we like one another; see if we want to work with each other; see if we can come to know each other, and be of help.

That is my offer, brother. I know I may not hear from you, so take care of yourself.

Compassionately yours,
Norm

Albee, G.W. *Mental health manpower trends.* New York: Basic Books, 1959.

Anthony, W.A., Buell, G.J., Sharratt, S., & Althoff, M.E. Efficacy of psychiatric rehabilitation. *Psychological Bulletin,* 1972, **78**, 447–456.

Appel, K. Constitutional law — Due process requires a standard of proof beyond a reasonable doubt for involuntary civil commitment. *Catholic University Law Review,* 1973, **23** (2), 409–416.

Arthur, A.Z. Diagnostic testing and the new alternatives. *Psychological Bulletin,* 1969, **72**: 183–192.

Ash, P. The reliability of psychiatric diagnosis. *Journal of Abnormal Social Psychology,* 1949, **44**, 272–276.

Bandura, A. *Principles of behavior modification.* New York: Holt, Rinehart & Winston, 1969.

Bazelon, D.L. Introduction in D.S. Burris, (Ed.), *The right to treatment: A symposium.* New York: Springer, 1969.

Beauchamp, T.L. Paternalism and biobehavioral control. *The Monist,* 1977, **60**, 62–80.

Bennett, C.C., Anderson, L.S., Cooper, S., Hassol, L., Klein, D.C., & Rosenblum, G. (Eds.). *Community psychology: A report of the Boston conference on the education of psychologists for community mental health.* Boston: Boston University Press, 1966.

Bernheim, H. *Suggestive therapeutics; A treatise on the nature and uses of hypnotism.* New York: London Book, 1947.

Bibliography

Bittner, E. Police discretion in emergency apprehension of mentally ill persons. In R.H. Price & B. Denner (Eds.), *The making of a mental patient.* New York: Holt, Rinehart, & Winston, 1973.

Bloch, S., & Reddaway, P. *Russia's political hospitals: The abuse of psychiatry in the Soviet Union.* London: V. Gollanez, 1977.

Bockoven, J.S. Moral treatment in American psychiatry. *Journal of Nervous and Mental Disease,* 1956, **124,** 167–183.

Braginsky, B.M., & Braginsky, D.D. Schizophrenia patients in the psychiatric interview: An experimental study of their effectiveness at manipulation. In R.H. Price & B. Denner (Eds.), *The making of a mental patient.* New York: Holt, Rinehart & Winston, 1973.

Braginsky, B.M., Braginsky, D.D., & Ring, K. *Methods of madness: The mental hospital as a last resort.* New York: Holt, Rinehart & Winston, 1969.

Braginsky, B.M., Grosse, M., & Ring, K. Controlling outcomes through impression management: An experimental study of the manipulative tactics of mental patients. In R.H. Price & B. Denner (Eds.), *The making of a mental patient.* New York: Holt, Rinehart & Winston, 1973.

Brill, N.Q., & Storrow, H.A. Social class and psychiatric treatment. In F. Riessman, J. Cohen, & A. Pearl (Eds.), *Mental health of the poor.* New York: Free Press, 1964.

Brown, B.S., Wienckowski, L.A., & Bivens, L.W. Psychosurgery: Perspective on a current issue (*U.S. Department of Health,*

Education & Welfare release). Washington, D.C.: U.S. Government Printing Office, 1973.

Burger, W.E. Psychiatrists, lawyers, and the courts, 28 Fed. Prob. 3, 7, 1964.

Buss, A.H. *Psychopathology*. New York: Wiley, 1966.

Caldwell, A.E. *Origins of psychopharmacology from CPZ to LSD*. Springfield, Ill.: Thomas, 1970.

Chu, F.D., & Trotter, S. *The mental health complex part I: Community mental health centers*. Washington, D.C.: Center for Study of Responsive Law, 1972.

Commission. *Report to the President from the President's commission on mental health*. Vol. I. Wash. D.C.: U.S. Government Printing Office, 1978.

Committee on Nomenclature and Statistics of the American Psychiatric Association. *Diagnostic and statistical manual: Mental disorders* (DSM-II). Washington, D.C.: American Psychiatric Association, 1968.

Cowen, E.L. Emergent approaches to mental health problems: An overview and directions for future work. In, E.L. Cowen, E.A. Gardner, & M. Zax (Eds.), *Emergent approaches to mental health problems*. New York: Appleton. Century-Crofts, 1967.

Cowen, E.L. Social and community interventions. *American Revue of Psychology* 1973, **24**, 423–472.

Deutsch, A. *The mentally ill in America: A history of their care and treatment from colonial times* (2d ed.). New York: Columbia University Press, 1949.

Dworkin, G. Paternalism. *The Monist*, 1972, **56**, 65.

Ennis, B.J. *Prisoners of psychiatry*. New York: Avon, 1972.

Ennis, B.J., & Emery, R.D. *The rights of mental patients*. (ACLU Handbook Series.) New York: Avon, 1978.

Ennis, B.J., & Siegel, L. *The rights of mental patients*. (ACLU Handbook Series.) New York: Avon, 1973.

Ennis, B.J., & Litwack, T.R. Psychiatry and the presumption of expertise: Flipping coins in the courtroom. *California Law Revue*, 1974, **62**, 693.

Erasmus, D. *Moriae encomium:* or *The praise of folly* (translated by W. Kennet). London: J. Wilford, 1735.

Erickson, M.H., Hershman, S., & Secter, I.I. *The practical application of medical and dental hypnosis*. New York: Julian Press, 1961.

Fairweather, G.W., (Ed.). *Social psychology in treating mental illness: An experimental approach.* New York: Wiley, 1964.

Feinberg, J. *Social philosophy.* New York: Prentice-Hall, 1973.

Finkel, N.J. *Mental illness and health: Its legacy, tensions, and changes.* New York: Macmillan, 1976.

Foucault, M. *Madness and civilization: A history of insanity in the age of reason.* New York: Vintage Books, 1973.

Frazer, Sir J.G. *The golden bough: A study in magic and religion.* New York: Macmillan, 1963.

Freud, S. The dynamics of transference (1912). In S. Freud, *Collected Papers* (Vol. II). London: Hogarth Press, 1953.

Freud, S. Recommendations for physicians on the psychoanalytic method of treatment (1912). In S. Freud, *Collected Papers* (Vol. II). London: Hogarth Press, 1953.

Freud, S. Further recommendations in the technique of psychoanalysis (1913). In S. Freud, *Collected Papers.* (Vol. II). London: Hogarth Press, 1953.

Freud, S. Analysis terminable and interminable (1937). In P. Rieff (Ed.), *Therapy and techniques.* New York: Collier, 1963.

Freud, S. *The interpretation of dreams* (translated by J. Strachey) (Discus Ed.). New York: Avon Books, 1967.

Freud, S. Project for a scientific psychology (1895). In J. Strachey (Ed.), *The standard edition of the complete psychological works of Sigmund Freud* (Vol. I.). London: Hogarth Press, 1974.

Friedman, P.R. Legal regulation of applied behavior analysis in mental institutions and prisons. *Arizona Law Revue.,* 1975, **17**, 39–104.

Gaylin, W. In the beginning: Helpless and dependent. In W. Gaylin, I. Glasser, S. Marcus, & D. Rothman (Eds.), *Doing good: The limits of benevolence.* New York: Pantheon, 1978.

Gaylin, W., Glasser, I., Marcus, S., & Rothman, D. *Doing good: The limits of benevolence.* New York: Pantheon Books, 1978.

Glasser, I. Prisoners of benevolence: Power versus liberty in the welfare state. In W. Gaylin, I. Glasser, S. Marcus, & D. Rothman (Eds.), *Doing good: The limits of benevolence.* New York: Pantheon, 1978.

Goffman, E. *The presentation of self in everyday life.* Garden City, N.Y.: Doubleday, 1959.

Goffman, E. *Asylums.* Garden City, N.Y.: Anchor, 1961.

Goffman, E. *Strategic interaction.* Philadelphia: University of Pennsylvania Press, 1969.

Goffman, E. The moral career of the mental patient. In R.H. Price & B. Denner (Eds.), *The making of a mental patient.* New York: Holt, Rinehart and Winston, 1973.

Goldberg, C. *Therapeutic partnership.* New York: Springer, 1977.

Goldfried, M.R., & Davison, G.C. *Clinical behavior therapy.* New York: Holt, Rinehart & Winston, 1976.

Goldhammer, H., & Marshall, A.W. *Psychosis and civilization.* New York: Free Press, 1949.

Gray, E. *A complete guide to the tarot.* New York: Bantam, 1970.

Gruenberg, E.M. The social breakdown syndrome—Some origins. *American Journal of Psychology, 123,* 12–120.

Gurin, G., Veroff, J., & Feld, S. *Americans view their mental health: A nationwide interview survey.* New York: Basic Books, 1960.

Haase, W. The role of socioeconomic class in examiner bias. In F. Riessman, J. Cohen, & A. Pearl (Eds.), *Mental health of the poor.* New York: Free Press, 1964.

Halleck, S.L. *The politics of therapy.* New York: Science House, 1971.

Hart, H.L.A. *Law, liberty, and morality.* Stanford, Calif.: Stanford University Press, 1963.

Hobbs, N. Mental health's third revolution. *American Journal of Orthopsychiatry,* 1964, **34,** 822–833.

Hobbs, N. Ethics in clinical psychology. In B.B. Wolman (Ed.), *Handbook of clinical psychology.* New York: McGraw-Hill, 1965.

Holland, J.G. Political implications of applying behavioral psychology. In R. Ulrich, T. Stachnik, & J. Mabry (Eds.), *Control of human behavior* (Vol. III). Glenview, Ill.: Scott, Foresman, 1974.

Hollingshead, B.B., & Redlich, F.C. *Social class and mental illness: A community study.* New York: Wiley, 1958.

Holzberg, J.D., Whiting, H.S., & Lowy, D.G. Chronic patients and a college companion program. In M. Zax & G. Stricker (Eds.), *The study of abnormal behavior: Selected readings* (2d ed.). New York: Macmillan, 1969.

Huxley, A.L. *Brave new world.* Garden City, N.Y.: Doubleday, 1932.

Huxley, A.L. *Brave new world revisited.* New York: Harper & Row, 1965.

Itard, J.M.G. *The wild boy of Aveyron.* New York: Meredith, 1962.

Joint Commission on Mental Illness and Health. *Action for mental health.* New York: Basic Books, 1961.

Jones, M. *The therapeutic community.* New York: Basic Books, 1953.

Kanfer, F.H., & Saslow, G. Behavioral diagnosis. In C.M. Franks (Ed.), *Behavior therapy: Appraisal and status.* New York: McGraw-Hill, 1969.

Kittrie, N.N. *The right to be different: Deviance and enforced therapy.* Baltimore: Johns Hopkins University Press, 1971.

Koenig, P. The problem that can't be tranquilized: 40,000 mental patients dumped in city neighborhoods. *The New York Times Magazine,* May 21, 1978.

Kozol, H., Boucher, R., & Garofalo, R. The diagnosis and treatment of dangerousness. *Crime and Delinquency,* 1972, **18,** 371–392.

Kreitman, N., Sainsbury, P., Morrissey, J., Towers, J., & Scrivener, J. The reliability of psychiatry assessment: An analysis. *Journal of Mental Science,* **107,** 887–908.

Leifer, R. The psychiatrist and tests of criminal responsibility. *American Psychologist,* 1964, **19,** 825–830. Copyright 1964 by the American Psychological Association. Reprinted by permission.

Livermore, J.M., Malmquist, C.P., & Meehl, P.E. On the justification for civil commitment. *University of Pennsylvania Law Revue,* 1968, **117,** 75–96.

London, P. *The modes and morals of psychotherapy.* New York: Holt, Rinehart & Winston, 1964.

Marcus, S. The brothers' keepers: An episode from English history. In W. Gaylin, I. Glasser, S. Marcus, & D. Rothman (Eds.), *Doing good: The limits of benevolence.* New York: Pantheon, 1978.

Meehl, P.E. Wanted – A good cookbook. *American Psychologist,* 1956, **11,** 263–272.

Menninger, K. *Theory of psychoanalytic technique.* New York: Harper & Row, 1958.

Mental Health Law Project. *Brief of Amici Curiae. Wyatt v. Aderholt,* Nov. 7, 1972.

Merriam-Webster. *Webster's seventh new collegiate dictionary.* Springfield, Mass.: Merriam, 1971.

Mill, J.S. *On liberty.* London: Watts (Thinker's Library), 1930.

Miller, D. Retrospective analysis of posthospital mental patients' worlds. *Journal of Health and Social Behavior,* 1967, **8,** 136–140.

Miller, D., & Schwartz, M. County Lunacy Commission hearings: Some observations of commitments to a state hospital. In R.H. Price & B. Denner (Eds.), *The making of a mental patient.* New York: Holt, Rinehart & Winston, 1973.

Monahan, J. The prevention of violence. In J. Monahan (Ed.), *Community mental health and the criminal justice system.* New York: Pergamon, 1976.

Moniz, E. How I came to perform prefrontal leucotomy. In T.S. Szasz (Ed.), *The age of madness: The history of involuntary mental hospitalization, presented in selected texts.* Garden City, N.Y.: Anchor Books, 1973.

Orwell, G. *1984: A novel.* New York: Harcourt, 1949.

Paul, G.L. Chronic mental patients: Current status – future direction. *Psychological Bulletin,* 1969, **71,** 81–94.

Philips, L., Breverman, I.K., & Zigler, E. Social competence and psychiatric diagnosis. *Journal of Abnormal Psychology,* 1966, **71,** 209–214.

Poser, E.G. The effect of therapist's training on group therapeutic outcome. *Journal of Consulting Psychology,* 1966, *30,* 283–289.

Price, R.H., & Denner, B. (Eds.) *The making of a mental patient.* New York: Holt, Rinehart Winston, 1973.

Rappaport, J. *Community psychology: Values, research, and action.* New York: Holt, Rinehart & Winston, 1977.

Rappaport, J., Chinsky, J.M., & Cowen, E.L. *Innovations in helping chronic patients: College students in a mental hospital.* New York: Academic Press, 1971.

Ray, I. *Medical jurisprudence of insanity.* Boston: Little & Brown, 1838.

Riessman, F., Cohen, J., & Pearl, A. *Mental health of the poor.* New York: Free Press, 1964.

Robinson, D.N. 1973. *Therapies: A clear and present danger. American Psychologist,* 1973, **28,** 129–33. Copyright 1973 by the American Psychological Association. Reprinted by permission.

Robinson, D. N. Harm, offense, and nuisance: Some first steps in the establishment of an ethics on treatment. *American Psychologist,* 1974, **29,** (4), 233–238. Copyright 1974 by the American Psychological Association. Reprinted by permission.

Robinson, D.N. *Autonomous man: Are reports of his death exaggerated?* Unpublished manuscript, 1976. (Available from the author, Georgetown University, Department of Psychology, Washington, D.C. 20057.)

Rothman, D. Introduction. In W. Gaylin, I. Glasser, S. Marcus, & D. Rothman (Eds.), *Doing good: The limits of benevolence.* New York: Pantheon, 1978.

Rothman, D. The state as parent: Social policy in the progressive era. In W. Gaylin, I. Glasser, S. Marcus, & D. Rothman (Eds.), *Doing good: The limits of benevolence.* New York: Pantheon, 1978.

Rubenstein, R., & Lasswell, H.D. *The sharing of power in a psychiatric hospital.* New Haven: Yale University Press, 1966.

Sanders, R. New manpower for mental hospital service. In E.L. Cowen, E.A. Gardner, & M. Zax (Eds.), *Emergent approaches to mental health problems.* New York: Appleton Century-Crofts, 1967.

Scheff, T.J. The societal reaction to deviance: Ascriptive elements in the psychiatric screening of mental patients in a midwestern state. In R.H. Price & B. Denner (Eds.), *The making of a mental patient.* New York: Holt, Rinehart & Winston, 1973.

Schmidt, H.O., & Fonda, C.P. The reliability of psychiatric diagnosis: A new look. *Journal of Abnormal Social Psychology,* 1956, **52**, 262–267.

Scholem, G.G. *Major trends in Jewish mysticism.* New York: Schocken Books, 1961.

Scott, E.P., & Ennis, B.J. *Motion for leave to file brief amicus curiae.* Washington, D.C.: Mental Health Law Project, 1975.

Singer, J. *Androgyny: Toward a new theory of sexuality.* Garden City, N.Y.: Anchor Books, 1977.

Skinner, B.F. *The behavior of organisms; an experimental analysis.* New York: Appleton-Century, 1938.

Skinner, B.F. *Beyond freedom and dignity.* New York: Bantam, 1971.

Smith, K., Pumphrey, M.W., & Hall, J.C. The "last straw": The decisive incident resulting in the request for hospitalization in 100 schizophrenic patients. In R.H. Price & B. Denner (Eds.), *The making of a mental patient.* New York: Holt, Rinehart & Winston, 1973.

Smith, W.G. A model for psychiatric diagnosis. *Archives of General Psychiatry,* 1966, **14**, 521–529.

Solzhenitsyn, A.I. *The Gulag Archipelago.* New York: Harper & Row, 1974.

Stone, A.A. *Mental health and the law: A system in transition.* Wash., D.C.: U.S. Government Printing Office, 1975.

Szasz T.S. *The myth of mental illness: Foundations of a theory of personal conduct.* New York: Hoeber-Harper, 1961.

Szasz, T.S. *Law, liberty, and psychiatry.* New York: Macmillan, 1963.

Szasz, T.J. *Ideology and insanity: Essays on the psychiatric dehumanization of man.* Garden City, N.Y.: Anchor Books, 1970.

Szasz, T.S. *The age of madness: The history of involuntary mental hospitalization, presented in selected texts.* Garden City, N.Y.: Anchor Books, 1973.

Task Panel, President's Commission on Mental Health. Mental health and human rights: Report of the task panel on legal and ethical issues. *Arizona Law Review,* 1978, *20,* 1, 49–174.

Thoresen, C.E., & Mahoney, M.J. *Behavioral self-control.* Monterey, Calif.: Brooks, Cole, 1974.

Torrey, E.F. *The death of psychiatry.* Radnor, Penn.: Chilton Book, 1974.

Towbin, A.P. Self-care unit: Some lessons in institutional power. *Journal of Consulting Clinical Psychology, 33,* 561–570.

Tuke, S. *Description of the Retreat, an institution near York, for insane persons of the Society of Friends.* London: Dawsons of Pall Mall, 1813.

Umbarger, C.C., Dalsimer, J.S., Morrison, A.P., & Breggin, P.R. *College students in mental hospitals.* New York: Grune & Stratton, 1962.

Urban, H.B., & Ford, D.H. Some historical and conceptual perspectives on psychotherapy and behavior change. In A.E. Bergin & S.L. Garfield (Eds.), *Handbook of psychotherapy and behavior change: An empirical analysis.* New York: Wiley, 1971.

Ward, C.H., Beck, A.T., Mendelson, M., Mock, J.E., & Erbaugh, J.K. The psychiatric nomenclature: Reasons for diagnostic disagreement. *Archives of General Psychiatry,* 1962. **7,** 198–205.

Wenger, D.L., & Fletcher, C.R. The effect of legal counsel on admissions to a state mental hospital: A confrontation of professions. In R.H. Price & B. Denner (Eds.), *The making of a mental patient.* New York: Holt, Rinehart & Winston, 1973.

Yarrow, M.R., Schwartz, C.G., Murphy, H.S., & Deasy, L.C. The psychological meaning of mental illness in the family. In R.H. Price & B. Denner (Eds.), *The making of a mental patient*. New York: Holt, Rinehart & Winston, 1973.

Zeydel, E.H. *The ship of fools by Sebastian Brant*. New York: Columbia University Press, 1944.

Zigler, E., & Philips, L. Psychiatric diagnosis: Critique. *Journal of Abnormal Social Psychology*, **63**, 607–618.

Zilboorg, G., & Henry, G.W. *A history of medical psychology*. New York: Norton, 1941.

Zusman, J. Some explanations of the changing appearance of psychotic patients. In R.H. Price & B. Denner (Eds.), *The making of a mental patient*. New York: Holt, Rinehart & Winston, 1973.

Index